FUTURESCAN™ 2014

Healthcare Trends and Implications 2014–2019

CONTENTS

T0206860

by Don Seymour

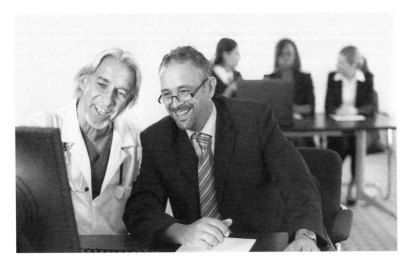

The title for this introduction derives from Sheldon B. Kopp's book, *If You Meet the Buddha on the Road, Kill Him!*

The premise, as you may surmise, is this: One can and should accept guidance, but one must always remember to seek his or her own "truth." Kopp (1972, 56) writes:

The most important things that each man must learn no one can teach him. Once he accepts this disappointment, he will be able to stop depending on . . . the guru who turns out to be just another struggling human being.

This wisdom applies to healthcare leaders in 2014. Consider the following:

- While some healthcare systems have been formed seemingly in the quest for scale for its own sake, others have prudently asked, "Scale to do what? How will it help us provide improved patient care?"
- Some healthcare organizations have rushed to sign up as Medicare accountable care organizations (ACOs). Others, some with well-established insurance company subsidiaries, have been more cautious, asking, "Are we prepared to assume actuarial risk for an attributed population with no lock into our network?"
- Marketing executives and some provider organizations see insurance exchanges as an immediate opportunity to increase volume. But their counterparts in other enterprises are skeptical. They ask, "How long will it actually take for half a dozen federal agencies (and a similar number at the state level) to implement this program? How long will it take to reach full enrollment?"
- Some leaders are reluctant to trade in their legacy IT systems

About the Author

Don Seymour, president of Don Seymour & Associates in Winchester, Massachusetts, has been a strategy adviser to hospital boards, CEOs, and medical staff leaders since 1979. A frequent presenter on subjects related to senior leadership in healthcare organizations, Seymour is on the faculties of the American College of Healthcare Executives and the Governance Institute. Additionally, he has made presentations to the American Hospital Association, numerous Fortune 100 companies, and a variety of other national, state, and regional groups. He has served as executive editor of *Futurescan™* since 2004. A past president of the Society for Healthcare Strategy & Market Development, he received its Award for Individual Professional Excellence in 2008.

for a platform that will truly support clinical integration and, in the long run, population health management. Others argue, "The time is now. The culture change alone may take ten years to get it right."
- While some leaders don't have the fortitude to battle for clinical integration and the employed physician model, others readily embrace the challenge: "It's the right thing to do, and it won't get easier if we wait."

Every pilgrim must chart his or her own journey to enlightenment; every healthcare provider must assess its own values, strengths, and limitations and then establish and pursue its own vision.

Enter *Futurescan*. Occasionally, readers ask, "How often have you been right?" It's a reasonable question. We strive always to be both accurate and correct, but we haven't kept score. Our editorial policy has focused more on raising issues that every provider faces on its journey and providing guidance and insight. We lack the wisdom and hubris to think that we are the Buddha; we are simply humble acolytes struggling with the challenges and opportunities inherent in the healthcare environment.

This year's edition of *Futurescan* continues in that tradition. We hope it enlightens your path as you delve into the following eight opinion pieces.

On coordinating care for population health: Forward-looking hospitals are engaging in challenging but necessary changes that promote population health. Whether improving the overall health of their population through better care coordination or working with community partners to improve the health of the broader community, hospitals are committing resources to promote population health. Participating in a health information exchange and sharing health data with other providers will allow hospitals to effectively address population health trends. Hospital and healthcare system leaders recognize that advancing population health will enable them to thrive in a value-based landscape. With strong collaborations, formal structures that enable care coordination, and the ability to leverage health data, hospitals can create population health initiatives that will lead to success in the evolving care environment.—Heather Jorna and Stephen A. Martin Jr., PhD

On measuring the success of population health: In the end, we must have a parallel strategy for keeping healthy people healthy and for managing the small percentage of patients who drive the vast majority of total costs in each of our local systems. Some vexing questions remain that we will have to answer in the next five years. For example, who owns the patient? Is it the attending physician, the ACO, the multispecialty group practice? Who is the real driver in improving the health of the population? Will this improvement all occur at the local, regional, or national level? How will we measure our success? Will the Triple Aim be relevant in five years, or will the Leading Health Indicators become the frontrunner?—David B. Nash, MD

On physician alignment: Although physician employment can simplify or eliminate many regulatory challenges, it is not a silver bullet for physician alignment. Because physician employment transactions can carry hefty capital investment costs and new practice expenses, large-scale employment is an impractical solution for many hospitals. Employment needs to be a carefully titrated ingredient in an overall physician alignment strategy. . . . Moving the dial on value will require expanded reliance on aligned primary care physicians, and you will need to face the financial headwinds that currently hamper progress. The creation of worthy financial incentives to fund and reward the transformation required to better manage populations at the primary care interface will be essential. Getting there will be hard, so start this work now.—Brian A. Nester, DO

On provider affiliations: The imperative for hospital leaders will be in honestly assessing and understanding how their organization can best serve its mission and the population entrusted to its care. Does the organization have the resources (financial, human, reputational, and intellectual) to be a controlling consolidator in this market, or is the organization better suited to play a more defined, participating role in the broader continuum? Does the organization truly understand how all of the fragmented components must come together and operate as a whole to achieve optimal performance against the metric of population health? Is the organization better suited to lead or to participate in a more defined role?—Mark Parrington, FACHE

On reimbursement and cost management: With such phenomenal changes in the healthcare market, hospital and healthcare leaders have no choice but to seek new opportunities for growth while also driving greater affordability for consumers and patients. We will have to reinvent ourselves and develop new markets and niche industries to meet our patients' expectations for quality care that is also affordable. It will not be the biggest among us who will survive; it will be the most creative and resourceful. Bringing value to patients—focusing on our mission and not our margins—will drive innovation that leads to sustainable business in healthcare. As hospital leaders, we can be the solution that America deserves.—Bernard J. Tyson

On information technology interoperability: Some leading organizations, small and large, have begun to derive benefits from coordinated care supported by robust IT infrastructure, such as single-source clinical solutions. "He who has the data will rule" will be the mantra of the future. More important, he who has the data and can turn it into meaningful information will be positioned for long-term success.—John P. Hoyt, FACHE, and Michael S. Wallace, FACHE

On equity of care: We do not have all the answers yet, but through the Call to Action and the Equity of Care platform, we are sharing resources and guides to help the field navigate toward high-quality care for all. To realize the goal of eliminating healthcare disparities, hospital leaders must believe that results can be achieved. The survey data highlight that this belief and commitment exist.—Richard J. Umbdenstock, FACHE

On efficiency: Employers and other payors will engage with narrow networks, high-performing networks, centers of excellence, or specialty units, sometimes through direct contracting. Employers will expect to benefit from increased efficiencies in the form of lower total charges and better results. For example, some savings may accrue to the employer and employee through faster patient recovery, fewer complications, fewer clinically unnecessary tests, and less rework. On the outpatient side, employers and other payors will want alternatives to emergency rooms, such as retail clinics. They will also want care options that keep people out of hospitals and away from hospital-based services. As hospitals try to provide a continuum of care to retain patients and capture revenue, employers and other payors will seek lower-cost alternatives.—Helen Darling 🅵🆂

Reference

Kopp, S.B. 1972. *If You Meet the Buddha on the Road, Kill Him!* New York: Bantam Books.

COORDINATING CARE TO PROVIDE EFFECTIVE POPULATION HEALTH MANAGEMENT

by Heather Jorna and Stephen A. Martin Jr., PhD

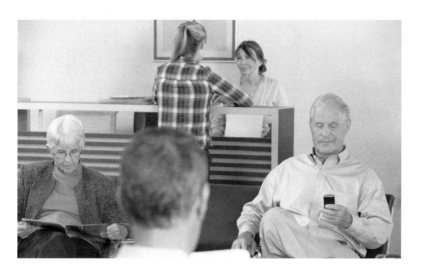

Hospitals and healthcare systems are focusing more attention on population health management as a tool to improve the health of their communities and patient bases.

Provisions in the Patient Protection and Affordable Care Act explicitly promote a population health approach by accelerating the transition to value-based payment models and by expanding access to healthcare services among newly insured populations. As hospitals increasingly are being held accountable for health outcomes, leaders need to proactively manage the health of populations beyond the acute care setting.

Population health management integrates public health principles into the healthcare delivery system. By focusing on upstream factors, such as health promotion and care coordination, population health management aims to deliver holistic healthcare that addresses a broad array of determinants of health to prevent chronic and acute disease. This approach to care significantly expands the traditional role of hospitals beyond their walls and into the community (HRET 2012; Stoto 2013).

The 2012 Annual Survey of Hospitals, conducted by the American Hospital Association, found that 98 percent of CEOs believe that hospitals need to investigate and implement population health management strategies. This task will require leaders to improve quality and patient safety, increase care coordination across the healthcare continuum, improve communication and information-sharing mechanisms, and expand preventive services and chronic disease management initiatives. To achieve these goals, hospital leaders are looking beyond traditional partnerships, such

About the Authors

Heather Jorna, MHSA, is the vice president of healthcare innovation at the American Hospital Association (AHA). In this role, she is responsible for leading the Hospitals in Pursuit of Excellence (HPOE) initiative, which is the AHA's strategic platform to accelerate performance improvement and support delivery system transformation in the nation's hospitals and health systems. Additionally, she is responsible for leading the AHA's Healthcare Transformation Fellowship, which is focused on building leadership skills in healthcare transformation including clinical integration, physician engagement, financial risk management, and population health management. Stephen A. Martin Jr., PhD, MPH, is the executive director of the Association for Community Health Improvement (ACHI) at the AHA. Previously, he served as the chief program officer of the Health Research & Educational Trust of the AHA, the health commissioner and chief operating officer of the Cook County Department of Public Health, and a senior executive member of the Cook County Health & Hospitals System. In addition, he has served as the secretary and treasurer of the Northern Illinois Public Health Consortium and the vice president of the Suburban Cook County Tuberculosis Sanitarium District.

as those with physicians and other clinicians, and are exploring relationships with community organizations, payors, and other health providers.

How likely is it that the following will be seen in your hospital's area by 2019?

Very Likely (%)	Somewhat Likely (%)	Somewhat Unlikely (%)	Very Unlikely (%)
43	27	18	12

Your hospital or health system **will control** a complete continuum of care in your service area through a variety of relationships.

21	32	29	19

Your hospital or health system will be a **noncontrolling** participant in a complete continuum of care in your service area through a variety of relationships.

51	42	7	1

Formal mechanisms will be in place in your service area to ensure seamless coordination across the care continuum (e.g., documented handoff processes for transition management, integrated health information portal).

55	37	8	1

A formal communication structure will be established between your hospital or system and community partners to promote population health (e.g., regular meetings, representation of community partners on board or planning committees).

Note: Percentages may not total to exactly 100% due to rounding.

What Practitioners Predict

Hospitals or health systems will participate in a continuum of care in their service area. A majority (70 percent) of survey respondents report that by 2019 it is likely that their hospital or health system will be in control of a complete continuum of care in their service area. Approximately half of the CEOs in the survey believe that their hospital or health system will be a noncontrolling partner in a care continuum by that time.

Formal mechanisms will ensure coordination across the continuum of care. Of CEOs surveyed, nearly 93 percent predict that mechanisms such as documented handoff processes and an integrated health information portal will be in place to ensure seamless coordination across the care continuum in their area by 2019.

Hospitals or health systems will work with community partners to promote population health. Almost all (92 percent) of the CEOs surveyed report it is likely that by 2019 a formal structure of communications, including regular meetings, will be established between their hospital or health system and community partners to promote population

How likely is it that the following will be seen in <u>your hospital</u> by 2019?

Very Likely (%)	Somewhat Likely (%)	Somewhat Unlikely (%)	Very Unlikely (%)
76		22	2 ◊

Your hospital will be partnering with community organizations to support population health management initiatives (e.g., community needs assessments, chronic disease management).

80		17	3 1

Your hospital will be participating in a health information exchange (HIE), which allows electronic sharing of health information among provider organizations.

12	42	31	15

Your hospital will require that its governing board have at least one member with population health expertise.

43	49	7	1

Your hospital will have effective measures of "population health" to support the community health improvement mandate.

Note: Percentages may not total to exactly 100% due to rounding.
◊ Less than 0.5%

health. Ninety-eight percent believe their organizations will work with community partners to promote population health management initiatives, such as community needs assessments or chronic disease management, by that time.

Hospitals or health systems will participate in a health information exchange (HIE). Almost all (97 percent) of the survey respondents predict that their organization will participate in an HIE that allows sharing of health information among providers by 2019.

Practitioners are divided about population health expertise on boards. Just over half of CEOs in the survey report it is likely that their hospital or health system will require that its governing board include at least one population health expert.

Population health measures will be established. Almost all CEOs surveyed (92 percent) predict that their hospitals or health systems will have effective measures of "population health" in place to support the community health mandate by 2019.

This year's *Futurescan* survey assessed the foundational elements necessary for population health management. The results reveal that within the next five years, a majority of hospitals will likely focus on (1) improving care coordination for their own patient base, while forming partnerships with community organizations, payors, and other health providers; (2) improving communication and care coordination mechanisms; and (3) sharing electronic health information to improve the health of populations.

Degree of Control Across the Care Continuum

Hospitals plan to work with other stakeholders to improve the patient experience across the care continuum, exercising various degrees of control by partnering with the community (AHA 2013; HRET 2012), affiliating with medical groups, and engaging and educating patients. Human capital and financial resources will factor into the decision whether a hospital will control the complete continuum of care or be a noncontrolling participant in the complete continuum of care.

Large hospitals and healthcare systems have increasingly aligned themselves with primary care and specialty practices; through these relationships, hospitals gain control of the continuum of care and use integrated electronic medical records to consolidate primary, specialty, and acute care encounters (Gamble 2012). Smaller and rural hospitals are more likely to collaborate with larger organizations than lead their own integration efforts (HRET 2013). Integrated delivery systems that already own facilities spanning a variety of health services (preventive, acute, post-acute, ancillary) have the resources and facilities to assume a greater degree of control and leadership in coordinating care across populations.

The *Futurescan* survey results support this trend: A majority of hospital leaders recognize the importance of population health strategies to achieve value-based care, expect some type of participation within the next five years, and are in the process of evaluating their role and degree of control in coordinating care.

Formal Mechanisms to Coordinate Across the Continuum of Care

Hospitals and healthcare systems are confident that formal care coordination structures that ensure seamless coordination across the care continuum, such as documented handoff processes and integrated health portals, will be in place by 2019. The formal mechanisms should optimize the use of health information across the continuum of care, resulting in fewer non-value-added treatments and better use of health resources to improve patient health and quality of care.

To become active participants in their own healthcare, patients must be engaged and given tools to manage their own health. Whether these tools include an integrated health portal, patient navigator, social worker, case manager, or community health worker, hospitals can adopt various mechanisms to drive patient involvement and accountability (AHA 2013).

Degree of Community Partnership

More and more hospitals are recognizing the value of addressing the health of populations beyond the traditional acute care setting. To successfully engage populations outside of their four walls, hospitals have to form community-based partnerships. These partnerships have the ability to (1) engage communities outside the hospital setting (HRET 2013), (2) expand the scope of the population served by the hospital, (3) align community needs with hospital offerings, and (4) address

upstream disease prevention in the community. Formal collaboration structures indicate a commitment to sustaining strong relationships with outside organizations. Post-acute care providers; government and commercial payors; employers; social and community services providers; public health agencies; local, state, and federal policy makers; physicians and other clinicians; and hospitals all play various roles in effectively engaging the patient in population health initiatives (AHA 2013). The specific groups with which a hospital collaborates are determined by the community's needs and the hospital's goals.

Participation in Health Information Exchanges

The *Futurescan* survey reveals important trends in electronic exchange of health data. The findings suggest that hospitals view information sharing as an important step toward better understanding and addressing the health status of populations. Participation in health information exchanges (HIEs) across the health system will be essential for monitoring and identifying population health trends, identifying opportunities for population health interventions, and predicting the impact of those interventions. Developing robust health information technology is essential for population health management because it will (1) allow providers to target at-risk populations in greatest need of services, (2) make the data actionable, and (3) generate alerts to providers about patient needs (Institute for Health Technology Transformation 2012). Although implementing an HIE presents myriad challenges, these systems will be crucial for managing population health.

Implications for Hospital Leaders

The aggregate *Futurescan* survey results indicate a strong commitment to population health advance-

Exhibit 1.1   Key Considerations by Hospital Type

Small/Rural Hospitals	• Take a more noncontrolling, network- or affiliation-type approach to population health initiatives because of their limited size and resources. • Can leverage their influence and relationships within communities to ensure successful programs.
Integrated Delivery Systems	• Have more opportunities to assume a coordinating role in population health initiatives with several community partners (e.g., a population health "integrator" role) because of their size and geographic reach. • Possess resources to engage in advocacy and policy efforts that promote better health and well-being.
Academic Medical Centers	• Face the challenge of aligning population health across their threefold mission—patient care, research, and medical education. • Often have high standing in their communities and can leverage their influence and prestige to engage partners.
Other	• Specialty hospitals can leverage their expertise to implement targeted population health programs in their communities (e.g., childhood obesity, heart health programs). • Faith-based hospitals can garner the support of religious organizations to supply volunteers for and financially support population health initiatives. • Stand-alone hospitals have fewer established affiliations and may therefore take a noncontrolling or networking-type approach to population health initiatives.

ment within the next five years. The degree and type of involvement a hospital will pursue will depend on the hospital's type, institutional culture, and competing priorities. Exhibit 1.1 lists key considerations for different hospital categories.

Conclusion

The *Futurescan* survey results support a paradigm shift toward population health management across the entire continuum of care within the next five years. Forward-looking hospitals are engaging in challenging but necessary changes that promote population health. Whether improving the overall health of their population through better care coordination or working with community partners to improve the health of the broader community, hospitals are committing resources to promote population health. Participating in an HIE and sharing health data with other providers will allow hospitals to effectively address population health trends.

Hospital and healthcare system leaders recognize that advancing population health will enable them to thrive in a value-based landscape. With strong collaborations, formal structures that enable care coordination, and the ability to leverage health data, hospitals can create population health initiatives that will lead to success in the evolving care environment. ▨

References

American Hospital Association (AHA). 2013. *Engaging Health Care Users: A Framework for Healthy Individuals and Communities.* Published January. Chicago: American Hospital Association. www.aha.org/research/cor/content/engaging_health_care_users.pdf.

———. 2012. "Annual Survey of Hospitals." Unpublished survey conducted November 2011 to January 2012. Data accessed July 2013.

Gamble, M. 2012. "Primary Care Strategy: The Most Important Decisions Hospitals Can Make." *Becker's Hospital Review.* Posted March 27. www.beckershospitalreview.com/hospital-physician-relationships/primary-care-strategy-the-most-important-decisions-hospitals-can-make.html.

Health Research & Educational Trust (HRET). 2013. *The Role of Small and Rural Hospitals and Care Systems in Effective Population Health Partnerships.* Published June. Chicago: Health Research & Educational Trust. www.hpoe. org/Reports-HPOE/The_Role_Small_Rural_Hospital_Effective_Population_Health_Partnership.pdf.

———. 2012. *Managing Population Health: The Role of the Hospital.* Published April. Chicago: Health Research & Educational Trust. www.hpoe.org/Reports-HPOE/managing_population_health.pdf.

Institute for Health Technology Transformation. 2012. *Population Health Management: A Roadmap for Provider-Based Automation in a New Era of Healthcare.* New York: Institute for Health Technology Transformation. http:// ihealthtran.com/pdf/PHMReport.pdf.

Stoto, M.A. 2013. *Population Health in the Affordable Care Act Era.* Published February 21. Washington, DC: AcademyHealth. www.academyhealth.org/files/AH2013pophealth.pdf.

PRACTICING POPULATION HEALTH MANAGEMENT AND MEASURING ITS SUCCESS

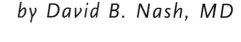

by David B. Nash, MD

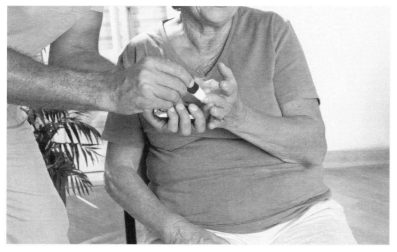

Americans are dying younger and living with a greater burden of disease than are residents of Slovenia and other less prosperous countries (Fineberg 2013; U.S. Burden of Disease Collaborators 2013).

Can the United States achieve improvements in the health of its population through reform provisions in the Affordable Care Act (ACA)? What is population health? What does it mean to "practice" population-based healthcare, and how do we measure its success? Finally, where is the movement toward population health going in the next five years?

About the Author

David B. Nash, MD, MBA, is the founding dean of the Jefferson School of Population Health on the campus of Thomas Jefferson University in Philadelphia, Pennsylvania. Dr. Nash is a board-certified internist and is internationally recognized for his work in outcomes management, medical staff development, and quality-of-care improvement. He has edited 22 books and published more than 100 scholarly articles in major journals. His national activities include membership on the boards of Main Line Health, the Care Continuum Alliance, Endo Health Solutions, and Humana. He is a consultant for organizations in the public and private sectors, including an appointment as chair of the technical advisory group of the Pennsylvania Healthcare Cost Containment Counsel. He is the editor-in-chief of four major national journals, including the *American Journal of Medical Quality*, *Population Health Management*, *Pharmacy and Therapeutics (P&T)*, and *American Health & Drug Benefits*. Through his writings, public appearances, and digital presence, his message reaches more than 100,000 persons every month.

Defining Population Health

The lack of agreement on any single operational definition of population health presents difficulties in interpreting current survey data and predicting the future. Population health can refer to "health outcomes and their distribution in a population. These outcomes are achieved by patterns of health determinants (such as medical care, public health, socioeconomic status, physical environment, individual behavior, and genetics) over the life course produced by policies and interventions at the individual and population levels" (Kindig 2007). This definition has been in our lexicon for at least three decades. Population health may also be viewed as the "aggregate health outcome of health-adjusted life expectancy (quantity and quality) of a group of individuals, in an economic framework that balances the relative marginal returns from the multiple determinants of health" (Kindig and Stoddart 2003). Others believe that population health is a sophisticated care delivery model that involves a systematic effort to assess the health needs of a target population and proactively provide services to maintain and improve the health of that population.

Population Health and Reform

Healthcare reform, through the ACA, features the implementation

How likely is it that the following will be seen in your hospital's area by 2019?

Very Likely (%)	Somewhat Likely (%)	Somewhat Unlikely (%)	Very Unlikely (%)
43	27	18	12

Your hospital or health system **will control** a complete continuum of care in your service area through a variety of relationships.

21	32	29	19

Your hospital or health system will be a **noncontrolling** participant in a complete continuum of care in your service area through a variety of relationships.

51	42	7	1

Formal mechanisms will be in place in your service area to ensure seamless coordination across the care continuum (e.g., documented handoff processes for transition management, integrated health information portal).

55	37	8	1

A formal communication structure will be established between your hospital or system and community partners to promote population health (e.g., regular meetings, representation of community partners on board or planning committees).

Note: Percentages may not total to exactly 100% due to rounding.

What Practitioners Predict

Hospitals or health systems will participate in a continuum of care in their service area. A majority (70 percent) of survey respondents report that by 2019 it is likely that their hospital or health system will be in control of a complete continuum of care in their service area. Approximately half of the CEOs in the survey believe that their hospital or health system will be a noncontrolling partner in a care continuum by that time.

Formal mechanisms will ensure coordination across the continuum of care. Of CEOs surveyed, nearly 93 percent predict that mechanisms such as documented handoff processes and an integrated health information portal will be in place to ensure seamless coordination across the care continuum in their area by 2019.

Hospitals or health systems will work with community partners to promote population health. Almost all (92 percent) of the CEOs surveyed report it is likely that by 2019 a formal structure of communications, including regular meetings, will be established between their hospital or health system and community partners to promote population

How likely is it that the following will be seen in <u>your hospital</u> by 2019?

Very Likely (%)	Somewhat Likely (%)	Somewhat Unlikely (%)	Very Unlikely (%)
76	22	2 ◊	

Your hospital will be partnering with community organizations to support population health management initiatives (e.g., community needs assessments, chronic disease management).

Very Likely (%)	Somewhat Likely (%)	Somewhat Unlikely (%)	Very Unlikely (%)
80	17	3	1

Your hospital will be participating in a health information exchange (HIE), which allows electronic sharing of health information among provider organizations.

Very Likely (%)	Somewhat Likely (%)	Somewhat Unlikely (%)	Very Unlikely (%)
12	42	31	15

Your hospital will require that its governing board have at least one member with population health expertise.

Very Likely (%)	Somewhat Likely (%)	Somewhat Unlikely (%)	Very Unlikely (%)
43	49	7	1

Your hospital will have effective measures of "population health" to support the community health improvement mandate.

Note: Percentages may not total to exactly 100% due to rounding.
◊ Less than 0.5%

health. Ninety-eight percent believe their organizations will work with community partners to promote population health management initiatives, such as community needs assessments or chronic disease management, by that time.

Hospitals or health systems will participate in a health information exchange (HIE). Almost all (97 percent) of the survey respondents predict that their organization will participate in an HIE that allows sharing of health information among providers by 2019.

Practitioners are divided about population health expertise on boards. Just over half of CEOs in the survey report it is likely that their hospital or health system will require that its governing board include at least one population health expert.

Population health measures will be established. Almost all CEOs surveyed (92 percent) predict that their hospitals or health systems will have effective measures of "population health" in place to support the community health mandate by 2019.

of two innovations in the delivery system to promote population health: patient-centered medical homes (PCMHs) and accountable care organizations (ACOs).

The PCMH model rests on the ability of a defined team to focus on the needs of the patient or family by coordinating a range of medical and social services. Among the challenges facing the PCMH movement is the fact that the evidentiary basis for the model's potential success does not yet exist! Work by leading investigators (e.g., Alexander et al. 2013) indicates that turning a typical primary care practice into a PCMH-designated center will require transformational change and a great deal of resources and organizational support that currently are not readily available.

ACOs, the other core reform component, rely on effective partnering among healthcare providers of all shapes and sizes—health systems, hospitals, clinics, physician practices, urgent care centers—to share responsibility for the health of a population and accountability for the cost of their care.

Practicing Population-Based Medicine

Practicing population health management is very different from the work of most health systems today. According to one industry analyst (Sg2 2013):

Organizations involved in population health must be concerned with all the determinants of health—environmental, social, economic and individual. Most of these factors fall outside the realm of traditional medicine, and there is no organization with the administrative, financial, and clinical resources to address them all. Therefore, PHM [population health management] must occur across a system of care—a broad network of alliances, partners and complementary organizations.

The essential components of such a comprehensive program might include, at a minimum, a care delivery infrastructure with advanced workforce models, innovative care delivery models (such as a PCMH), and a robust primary care network. Another key component is a technology infrastructure that will enable providers to risk-stratify the patients within a population and readily share information about both processes and outcomes. Finally, practicing population health management requires a culture of innovation, effective physician leadership, and risk-contracting payment models (Sg2 2013).

Futurescan Survey Results

Let's examine the current *Futurescan* survey results in light of the challenges in defining, organizing, and implementing systems to support population health management.

Notably, a majority (70 percent) of survey respondents report that in the next five years their hospital or health system will likely be in control of a complete continuum of care in their service area. Personally, I find this prediction implausible because of all of the inherent challenges in managing a coordinated continuum of care. Another surprising result is that, of the CEOs surveyed, nearly 93 percent predict that mechanisms, such as documented handoff processes and integrated health information portals, will be in place to ensure seamless coordination of care across the continuum in the next five years. All of the available evidence indicates that implementation of such mechanisms will be a nearly insurmountable challenge (DesRoches et al. 2013).

I was heartened to learn that 92 percent of the CEOs surveyed believe that, within the next five years, they will create a formal structure of communication, including regular meetings between their

hospitals and local community partners, to promote population health.

Finally, practitioners remain sharply divided on population health expertise at the governance level. I was surprised that more than half of CEOs in the survey report that their hospital will likely require at least one population health expert on its governance board. Where will this expertise come from, and how will boards find these persons and bring them into the fold? As the dean of the only school of population health in the nation, I certainly hope that some of our emerging leaders will fill this role!

Measuring Success

How will we measure the success of the population health movement? Here, I am in complete agreement with the majority of CEOs who predict that hospitals and health systems will have effective measures of population health in place to support the community health mandate by 2019.

Let's take a broader look at measuring population health. Some experts (e.g., Stiefel and Nolan 2013) believe that greater attention to achieving the so-called Triple Aim of the Institute for Healthcare Improvement (health of the population, individual experience of care, and per capita cost) will advance our ability to measure the health of the population.

As organizations move from strategy to execution, they will need better measures for each dimension of the Triple Aim. Population health measures might include years of potential life lost, life expectancy, and standardized mortality rates. For measuring the experience of care, Consumer Assessment of Healthcare Providers and Systems (CAHPS) data might provide benchmarks. Finally, for per capita cost, measures such as the total cost per population member per month and certain hospital and emergency department utilization rates might be appropriate.

In a recent report, the Institute of Medicine made recommendations about quality measures for population health (IOM 2013). This watershed report links major public health outcomes, such as the Leading Health Indicators (selected key objectives of the Healthy People 2020 agenda), to population health outcomes, such as better care coordination and reduction in waste. Perhaps the IOM report, combined with work on the Triple Aim, might help formulate measures of population health in the near future.

Implications for Hospital Leaders

Stepping into population health management will present a series of challenges to most hospitals and health systems. These challenges can be addressed in several stages (Sg2 2013). The first stage builds the basic foundation for population health management by focusing on traditional cost and quality measures, such as unnecessary emergency department visits or readmission rates by disease and source of admission. Potentially avoidable admission rates or admissions per 1,000 measures of a defined population could be other first-stage measures. This first stage can be implemented right now.

The second stage might deploy available first-generation population health metrics, such as those for diabetic adults with a hemoglobin A1C level greater than 8 percent or adults with a body mass index greater than 25 who have a documented follow-up plan. How about screening rates for colorectal and breast cancer, tobacco use, and depression? We can experiment and begin an early organizational transformation using some of these off-the-shelf population health metrics.

The next stage might focus on our ability to deploy core population health management capabilities and to master longitudinal metrics, such as managing a population in a per-member per-month payment scheme or obtaining detailed information about out-of-network utilization and true resource utilization in both the inpatient and outpatient settings. We should study how much we are really spending on certain chronic conditions and where that spending occurs (in the hospital versus in the ambulatory setting). And then we might be ready for the final stage, which would be to refine population-wide quality-of-life and functional assessments and customized measures of the effectiveness of certain interventions.

We need to create a checklist for population health management (Nash et al. 2011), which would include

- implementing health risk assessments,
- promoting prevention and wellness programs,
- building PCMHs,
- linking with local retail clinics or building our own,
- partnering with managed care companies,
- establishing true electronic registries so that we can track patient populations, and
- implementing physician leadership training in all areas relevant to population health management.

In the end, we must have a parallel strategy for keeping healthy people healthy and for managing the small percentage of patients who drive the vast majority of total costs in each of our local systems.

Some vexing questions remain that we will have to answer in the next five years. For example, who owns the patient? Is it the attending physician, the ACO, the multispecialty group practice? Who is the real driver in improving the health of the population? Will this improvement all occur at the local, regional, or national level? How will we measure our success? Will the Triple Aim be relevant in five years, or will the Leading Health Indicators become the front-runner?

There is no excuse for Americans dying younger and living with more illness than the residents of other nations. For a country that spends more on healthcare than any other country on the planet (Kumar and Nash 2011), we all should demand better! ▣

References

Alexander, J.A., G.R. Cohen, C.G. Wise, and L.A. Green. 2013. "The Policy Context of Patient Centered Medical Homes: Perspectives of Primary Care Providers." *Journal of General Internal Medicine* 28 (1): 147–53.

DesRoches, C.M., A.M. Audet, M. Painter, and K. Donelan. 2013. "Meeting Meaningful Use Criteria and Managing Patient Populations: A National Survey of Practicing Physicians." *Annals of Internal Medicine* 158 (11): 791–99.

Fineberg, H.V. 2013. "The State of Health in the United States." *Journal of the American Medical Association* 310 (6): 585–86.

Institute of Medicine (IOM). 2013. *Toward Quality Measures for Population Health and the Leading Health Indicators.* Washington, DC: National Academies Press.

Kindig, D.A. 2007. "Understanding Population Health Terminology." *Milbank Quarterly* 85 (1): 139–61.

Kindig, D.A., and G. Stoddart. 2003. "What Is Population Health?" *American Journal of Public Health* 93 (3): 380–83.

Kumar S., and D.B. Nash. 2011. *Demand Better! Revive Our Broken Healthcare System.* Bozeman, MT: Second River Healthcare Press.

Nash, D.B., J. Reifsnyder, R. Fabius, and V.P. Pracilio. 2011. *Population Health: Creating a Culture of Wellness.* Sudbury, MA: Jones & Bartlett Learning.

Sg2. 2013. *Population Health Management.* White paper. Skokie, IL: Sg2. www.sg2.com.

Stiefel, M., and K. Nolan. 2013. "Measuring the Triple Aim: A Call for Action." *Population Health Management* 16 (4): 219–20.

U.S. Burden of Disease Collaborators. "The State of US Health, 1990–2010: Burden of Diseases, Injuries, and Risk Factors." *Journal of the American Medical Association* 310 (6): 591–608.

PHYSICIAN–HOSPITAL ALIGNMENT: AN ESSENTIAL INGREDIENT IN VALUE PRODUCTION

by Brian A. Nester, DO

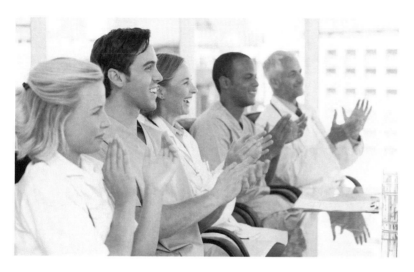

Given the Institute of Medicine's estimate that roughly 30 percent of healthcare spending is wasteful, an opportunity exists to deliver appropriate and high-quality care to more people at a lower cost in our respective communities (IOM 2012).

Value production in healthcare—that is, creating access to affordable and high-quality care—addresses unjustifiable variations and outright failures in care delivery. Implementing value production, however, necessitates a highly aligned ethical, financial, and clinical compact between hospital and physician providers to efficiently and effectively address the needs of the populations they serve—together.

Trends

The economic feasibility of an independent medical practice will continue to evaporate. The aggregate impact of declining reimbursement, growing practice overhead, mounting regulatory mandates, and student loan debt is escalating physicians' pessimism about the economic feasibility of working in private practice (Beaulieu 2012; Harris 2010; Jackson Healthcare 2013). Hospitals will continue to step in and, by employing physicians and providing practice subsidies, develop an aligned physician workforce—an essential ingredient for remaining competitive and aggregating attributable lives for the future game of accountable care. The law of supply and demand will generally favor physician income, with small to modest increases in the coming years (especially in primary care and hospital-employed models). The question is, will these income increases be enough—and in the

About the Author

Brian A. Nester, DO, MS, MBA, CPE, FACOEP, is currently chief strategy officer at Lehigh Valley Health Network (LVHN) in Allentown, Pennsylvania. He is charged with aligning LVHN's business development assets with evolving population health management competencies and insurance sophistication in creating new partnerships and structures to facilitate LVHN's transformation into an accountable care organization. From 2003 to 2011, as senior vice president for physician–hospital network development, he worked to develop LVHN's aligned physician base, which includes more than 600 employed physicians and more than 200 independent physicians in a variety of contractual arrangements. He serves as chairman of the board of the Lehigh Valley Physician Hospital Organization and is a member of the board of the Hospital and Health System of Pennsylvania (HAP), serving as chair of the physician advisory task force for HAP. He speaks nationally on issues related to physician integration and business development and speaks regularly at Columbia University's Graduate School of Business and Mailman School of Public Health on issues related to healthcare reform and strategy. He is an emergency physician, a Certified Physician Executive (CPE) endorsed by the American College of Physician Executives, and a member of the Society for Healthcare Strategy & Market Development.

How likely is it that the following will be seen in your hospital's area by 2019?

Very Likely (%)	Somewhat Likely (%)	Somewhat Unlikely (%)	Very Unlikely (%)
44	40	14	2

Fifty percent or more of the primary care physician workforce in your community will be committed to accepting **new** Medicare patients in their practices.

40	45	13	1

Most primary care physicians in your community will support patient-centered medical homes as the best way to deliver value-based care.

How likely is it that the following will be seen in <u>your hospital</u> by 2019?

	Very Likely (%)	Somewhat Likely (%)	Somewhat Unlikely (%)	Very Unlikely (%)
ACHE	47	23	21	9
SHSMD	60	28	10	2
Both	51	24	18	7

Your hospital and physicians in your community will have established a physician–hospital organization (PHO), where physicians and your hospital join to negotiate and obtain contracts with insurance plans and employers.

75	22	2	◊

There will be increased cooperation between your hospital and physicians in your community.

60	31	8	1

Your hospital will have increased resources for physician leadership training.

64	32	4	◊

Hospital and physician incentives to deliver value-based care (e.g., reducing medical costs, improving HCAHPS outcomes) will be aligned.

Note: Percentages may not total to exactly 100% due to rounding.

◊ Less than 0.5%

Primary care physicians will accept new Medicare patients. Most (nearly 84 percent) of the practitioners surveyed think it likely that over half of the primary care physicians in their area will be committed to accepting new Medicare patients in their practices by 2019.

Primary care physicians will support patient-centered medical homes (PCMHs). Of the CEOs surveyed, more than 85 percent report it is likely that most primary care physicians will support patient-centered medical homes as the best way to deliver value-based care by 2019.

Hospitals will participate in physician–hospital organizations. Seventy percent of ACHE respondents and 88 percent of SHSMD respondents believe that by 2019 their hospital and physicians in their area will have established physician–hospital organizations (PHOs), where physicians and hospitals together negotiate and obtain contracts with insurance plans and employers.

Cooperation between physicians and hospitals will increase. Nearly all (97 percent) of the respondents report that cooperation between their hospitals and physicians in their area is likely to increase by 2019.

Investment in physician leadership training will increase. Almost all (91 percent) of the CEOs surveyed predict that their hospital will increase resources for physician leadership training by 2019.

Value-based care incentives will be aligned. Almost all (96 percent) of the survey respondents predict that by 2019 incentives for their hospital and its associated physicians to deliver value-based care will be aligned.

right formulation—to incentivize and ignite population-focused care transformation?

Administrative and billing functions will become increasingly complex for office practices.
Managing administrative complexity demands a variety of resources, and office staff can spend as many as 20 hours per week per physician on billing-related matters alone (Morra et al. 2011; Sakowski et al. 2009). Some physicians will reluctantly make adjustments to their practices to address billing issues— for example, seeing fewer patients, excluding Medicaid patients, or limiting access for Medicare patients (Physicians Foundation 2012). Many physicians, however, will leave their practices and seek employment by a hospital or health system. While estimates of physician employment vary, more than 75 percent of physicians could be employed by hospitals or other healthcare companies before the end of this decade (Accenture 2011; Kocher and Sahni 2011).

Competition for patients in the ambulatory space will become fierce as alternative providers and new care outlets emerge.
Urgent care centers, minute clinics, and stand-alone retail emergency rooms are among the alternative providers offering ready access and price-sensitive solutions to consumers (Mehrotra and Lave 2012). Although these options provide relief to a busy physician practice, they can also fragment care if treatment is not adequately communicated. The rapid segmentation of ambulatory services around convenience and service will continue, and physician practices and hospitals will need to transform their operations to compete or otherwise simply step aside (Cassel 2012; Watson 2013).

Physicians will meet current challenges. Transforming the operational focus of a traditional medical practice to one that emphasizes access, service, wellness, and outcomes is more than just an objective—it's a business model. To this end, large primary care and

multispecialty groups are organizing, and some independent practice associations and physician–hospital organizations are reorganizing, to meet the accountable care challenge. Physician group accountable care organizations (ACOs) now outnumber health system ACOs (Hertz 2013; Muhlestein 2013). Whether with Medicare or a commercial payor, physicians are entering accountable care contracts, which often target lower inpatient utilization (Zigmond 2013). If hospitals are not involved in these accountable care conversations, they will remain on the outside as progressive physicians independently contribute to the maturation of the accountable care movement.

Challenges will disproportionately impact primary care providers.
Primary care providers (PCPs) have struggled for decades to promote population health—an unpopular movement until now. Although quality incentives and pay-for-performance strategies are gaining strength, their financial impact

on PCPs is minuscule. What's more, the reporting obligations are burdensome for PCPs, who bear a disproportionate responsibility for driving value-based care delivery improvements (Catalyst for Payment Reform 2013; Fiegl 2013). Waiting for a federal policy to dictate local market strategies for sparking PCP engagement and assisting them in value production is not a prudent course.

Implications for Hospital Leaders

Hospitals must integrate more fully with both employed and independent physicians to address the financial challenges of a new healthcare economy. The future will be characterized by value-based reimbursement and declining

opportunities for revenue maximization. Limited pilots between hospitals and physicians are important but will simply not suffice—it's time to pick your physician partners and transform. The following tactics can support successful physician integration efforts.

Assess your physician community. Seek and identify physician leaders. Whether they are clinicians who engender trust among referring physicians or physician practice leaders who provide direction to the medical community—know who they are.

Listen to your physician leaders. Engage physician leaders on the shared responsibility you both have for a common community. Strap yourself in for the ride and don't

be surprised if those conversations cause you to scale back your initial expectations for physician engagement in patient-centered medical homes or the acceptance of new Medicare patients. Active listening is a first step in the right direction.

Recognize that words matter. In alignment conversations, a shared vision is key. Meaningful engagement will likely not come if physicians think hospitals are asking them to "integrate into" or "align with" hospital objectives.

Be more transparent with your physician leaders. Transparency requires sharing timely reports on hospital quality and financial performance, the objective being shared responsibility. Physician

Exhibit 3.1 Correlation of Contractual Mechanisms with Operational Risk and Alignment

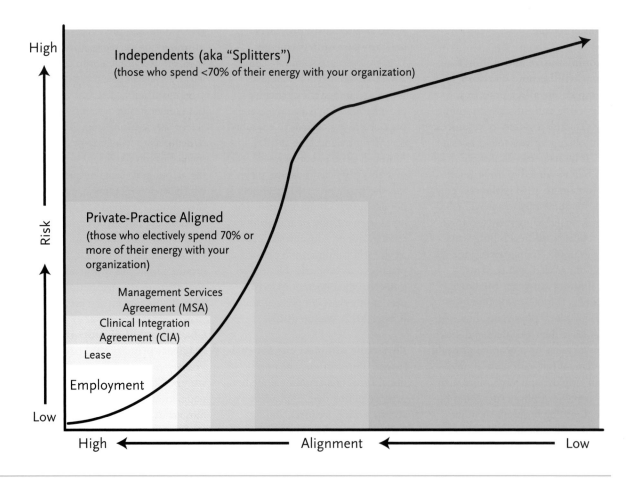

leaders should have ready access to hospital leadership (including the CEO), especially as it relates to operational issues that affect patient care and provider efficiency.

Get shared-risk expectations on the table. An honestly brokered and respectful conversation (or joint educational process) about risk tolerance in accountable care may expedite and strengthen your organization's bond with important physician constituencies. Initiating dialogue through a new or revitalized physician–hospital organization, independent practice association, or local medical society chapter may yield a healthy conversation about risk expectations and any potential split on shared savings.

Be open to a variety of physician–hospital business agreements. A wide range of contractual agreements exists, including management or purchased service agreements, clinical integration agreements, ancillary joint ventures, and practice leases. My experience with different physician arrangements drives the intuition that operational alignment generally increases and operational risk generally decreases (for both hospitals and physicians) as the substance of the arrangement moves closer to employment of physicians by the hospital or health system (see Exhibit 3.1). Providing contractual alternatives allows movement along this alignment axis, because one size does not fit all. Given the regulatory climate and the complexity of physician–hospital agreements, hospital leaders are wise to involve experienced transaction consultants.

Weigh physician employment against other business agreements. Although physician employment can simplify or eliminate many regulatory challenges, it is not a silver bullet for physician alignment. Because physician employment transactions can carry hefty capital investment costs and new practice expenses, large-scale employment is an impractical solution for many hospitals. Employment needs to be a carefully titrated ingredient in an overall physician alignment strategy.

Make primary care a priority. Moving the dial on value will require expanded reliance on aligned PCPs, and you will need to face the financial headwinds that currently hamper progress. The creation of worthy financial incentives to fund and reward the transformation required to better manage populations at the primary care interface will be essential. Getting there will be hard, so start this work now.

Conclusion

The transformation of our healthcare economy from fee-for-service to fee-for-value is a daunting endeavor, demanding macro-level maneuvers such as payment innovation, industry consolidation, and leveraging big data. In the end, the essential translation of value-based care will require newly focused micro-interactions between providers and patients. Consequently, implementing value production (creating access to affordable and high-quality care) in most communities will take place only through an aligned commitment by hospitals and physicians to serve a common patient population. FS

References

Accenture. 2011. *Clinical Transformation: Dramatic Changes as Physician Employment Grows*. Published March 28. www.accenture.com/us-en/Pages/insight-clinical-transformation-physician-employment-grows.aspx.

Beaulieu, D. 2012. "One-Quarter of Small Practices Eyeing Closure." FiercePracticeManagement. Published July 4. www.fiercepracticemanagement.com/story/one-quarter-small-practices-eyeing-closure/2012-07-04.

Cassel, C.K. 2012. "Retail Clinics and Drugstore Medicine." *Journal of the American Medical Association* 307 (20): 2151–52.

Catalyst for Payment Reform. 2013. *National Scorecard on Payment Reform*. Published March 26. www.catalyzepaymentreform.org/images/documents/NationalScorecard.pdf.

Fiegl, C. 2013. "Medicare Proposes Doctor Pay for Complex Chronic Care Management." *American Medical News*. Posted July 22. www.amednews.com/article/20130722.

Harris, G. 2010. "More Doctors Giving Up Private Practices." *New York Times*, March 25. www.nytimes.com/2010/03/26/health/policy/26docs.html.

Hertz, B.T. 2013. "A Look at Physician-Led ACOs: What's Driving Them, and Where They're Headed." *Medical Economics.* Published June 10. http://medicaleconomics.modernmedicine.com/medical-economics/news/look-physician-led-acos-whats-driving-them-and-where-theyre-headed.

Institute of Medicine (IOM). 2012. *Best Care at Lower Cost: The Path to Continuously Learning Health Care in America.* Washington, DC: National Academies Press.

Jackson Healthcare. 2013. *Filling the Void: 2013 Physician Outlook and Practice Trends.* eBook. www.jacksonhealthcare.com/media/191888/2013physiciantrends-void_ebk0513.pdf.

Kocher R., and N.R. Sahni. 2011. "Hospitals' Race to Employ Physicians —The Logic Behind a Money-Losing Proposition." *New England Journal of Medicine* 364 (19): 1790–93.

Mehrotra, A., and J.R. Lave. 2012. "Visits to Retail Clinics Grew Fourfold from 2007 to 2009, Although Their Share of Overall Outpatient Visits Remains Low." *Health Affairs* 31 (9): 2123–29.

Morra D., S. Nicholson, W. Levinson, D.N. Gans, T. Hammons, and L.P. Casalino. 2011. "US Physician Practices Versus Canadians: Spending Nearly Four Times as Much Money Interacting with Payers." *Health Affairs* 30 (8): 1443–50.

Muhlestein, D. 2013. "Continued Growth of Public and Private Accountable Care Organizations." *Health Affairs Blog.* Posted February 19. http://healthaffairs.org/blog/2013/02/19/continued-growth-of-public-and-private-accountable-care-organizations/.

Physicians Foundation. 2012. *A Survey of America's Physicians: Practice Patterns and Perspectives.* Published September 21. www.physiciansfoundation.org/uploads/default/Physicians_Foundation_2012_Biennial_Survey.pdf.

Sakowski J.A., J.G. Kahn, R.G. Kronick, J.M. Newman, and H.S. Luft. 2009. "Peering into the Black Box: Billing and Insurance Activities in a Medical Group." *Health Affairs* 28 (4): 544–54.

Watson, S. 2013. "More Americans Using Retail Health Clinics." *Harvard Health Blog.* Posted May 10. www.health.harvard.edu/blog/more-americans-using-retail-health-clinics-201305106189.

Zigmond, J. 2013. "Why One Medicare Pioneer ACO Succeeded in Saving Money." *ModernHealthcare.com.* Published July 16. www.modernhealthcare.com/article/20130716/NEWS/307169946.

HEALTHCARE REFORM AND INCORPORATING MISSION, VALUES, AND CULTURE IN PROVIDER AFFILIATIONS

by Mark Parrington, FACHE

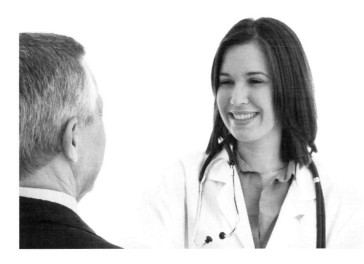

Scott Serota opened his *Futurescan 2013* essay on insurer–provider integration with the statement:

"A central barrier to creating a healthcare system that provides Americans with the best, most affordable care possible is the high degree of fragmentation that traditionally has existed among the many parties involved in delivering, managing, financing, and receiving that care" (Serota 2013). Healthcare reform focuses on removing that central barrier—the high degree of fragmentation. Reform's emphasis on both integrated delivery of care and population health suggests that these two components will come together to respond more effectively to the needs of the whole by reducing the degree of fragmentation.

The Wave of Mergers and Acquisitions

Due largely to healthcare reform initiatives, changing healthcare market imperatives and increasing economic pressures continue to drive the consolidation of healthcare systems and hospitals. A perceived need for greater scale to accommodate the new demands on the delivery system also underlies this consolidation. Today's trends are therefore not surprising—hospital and health system mergers and acquisitions (M&As) have doubled over the past three years, and the number of significant M&As (involving $1 billion or more) has increased (Booz & Company 2013). Within the M&A context, a range of structures and arrangements are available, including loose coalitions and collaborations, transfers of minority interests, joint operating agreements, and the ultimate in "integrating relationships"—a full merger or acquisition.

According to a recent report, "virtually every hospital and health

About the Author

Mark Parrington, FACHE, is vice president of strategic transactions and development at Catholic Health Initiatives (CHI), a national healthcare delivery system based in Englewood, Colorado. He has more than 35 years of diversified and highly effective experience in strategic planning, marketing, and business development with an emphasis on the planning and development of integrated healthcare delivery systems. Prior to joining CHI in 2006, Parrington held senior strategy and business development executive positions at Centegra Health System in Crystal Lake, Illinois; The Cleveland Clinic Health System–Western Region in Cleveland, Ohio; and Mercy in St. Louis, Missouri, and he served for 15 years as a member of the founding senior management team at Sutter Health in Sacramento, California. He has served on many professional, corporate, and community boards of directors, including currently on the board of directors of the AHA's Society for Healthcare Strategy & Market Development, where he serves as president-elect. Parrington has addressed numerous national audiences on current healthcare topics and has authored and coauthored a number of articles throughout his career.

system will be touched by the new wave of deals, as an acquirer, an acquired company, or an organization contemplating such moves. Even if a hospital or health system

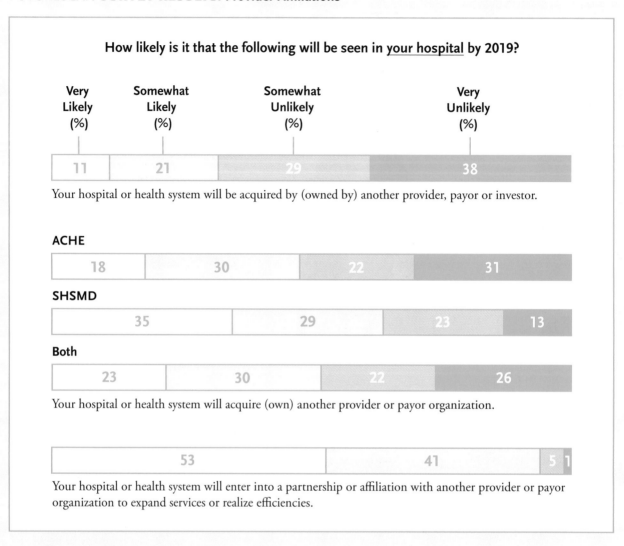

How likely is it that the following will be seen in <u>your hospital</u> by 2019?

Very Likely (%)	Somewhat Likely (%)	Somewhat Unlikely (%)	Very Unlikely (%)
11	21	29	38

Your hospital or health system will be acquired by (owned by) another provider, payor or investor.

ACHE

| 18 | 30 | 22 | 31 |

SHSMD

| 35 | 29 | 23 | 13 |

Both

| 23 | 30 | 22 | 26 |

Your hospital or health system will acquire (own) another provider or payor organization.

| 53 | 41 | 5 | 1 |

Your hospital or health system will enter into a partnership or affiliation with another provider or payor organization to expand services or realize efficiencies.

Note: Percentages may not total to exactly 100% due to rounding.

What Practitioners Predict

Providers are divided about hospital acquisitions. Two-thirds of CEOs surveyed think it unlikely that their hospital or health system will be acquired by another provider, payor, or investor between now and 2019. Forty-eight percent of ACHE respondents and 64 percent of SHSMD respondents consider it likely that their hospital or system will acquire another provider or payor organization over the next five years.

Partnerships between providers will increase. Most (94 percent) of the survey respondents predict that by 2019 their hospital or health system will enter into affiliations or partnerships with other providers or payor organizations, either to expand their services or to realize efficiencies.

does not intend to pursue M&A activity, or wants to remain independent, it must have a plan in place to thoughtfully consider M&A opportunities and offers as they arise, to effectively navigate the changing post-reform landscape" (Booz & Company 2013).

Futurescan Survey Results

This year's *Futurescan* survey results shed light on shifting provider affiliations and reveal what appears to be either conflicting data or a degree of uncertainty in the healthcare delivery marketplace. Fully two-thirds of CEOs think it unlikely that their hospital or health system will be acquired between now and 2019, while approximately half consider it likely that they will acquire another provider or payor within the next five years.

In response to a slightly different question in the Efficiency category of the survey (see pages 42–43), two-thirds of CEOs reported that their organization will likely merge with another to reduce operating costs. So, the survey responses appear to reflect a dichotomy. Two-thirds find it unlikely that they will be acquired, yet two-thirds think it likely that they will merge. Here we see respondents making a distinction between *acquire* and *merge* and their respective degrees of control— "owned by" versus "partnership with."

In the Population Health category of the survey (see page 6), 70 percent of CEOs believe their organization will, within the next five years, control a complete continuum of care through a variety of relationships, while 53 percent think their hospital or health system will be a noncontrolling participant in such a continuum.

Perhaps the most telling survey finding is that 94 percent of CEOs predict that by 2019, their organizations will enter into affiliations or partnerships with other provider or payor organizations, either to expand their services or to realize efficiencies.

These trends will play themselves out over the next five years across a variety of markets and through a variety of models, within time frames that will differ according to how quickly each market evolves. Any number of organizations will assume controlling positions, and any number will thrive as noncontrolling participants. But ultimately, the vast majority expect to be in relationships different from those they are in today.

Implications for Hospital Leaders

The imperative for hospital leaders will be in honestly assessing and understanding how their organization can best serve its mission and the population entrusted to its care. Does the organization have the resources (financial, human, reputational, and intellectual) to be a controlling consolidator in this market, or is the organization better suited to play a more defined, participating role in the broader continuum? Does the organization truly understand how all of the fragmented components must come together and operate as a whole to achieve optimal performance against the metric of population health? Is the organization better suited to lead or to participate in a more defined role?

While the survey may present some uncertainty as to who will control and who will be noncontrolling participants, a number of points are clear. No single model will predominate, but rather an array of models will emerge for different markets at different times. These models may evolve over time. A variety of relationships will accommodate the diverse roles required to achieve the goals of healthcare reform within the construct of population health. These models and relationships will reflect differences in the degree of control, ranging from "owned by" to "in partnership with." And in the final accounting, the success of the venture may rest not on a given structure or the strengths and resources of the participants but rather on how ably the mission, values, and cultures of the participants are blended.

The language of mission statements and the articulation of values are often similar from organization to organization. The key distinction lies in how these missions and values are lived within organizations— their culture. Is decision making top-down, or is it collaborative and inclusive? Is the organization flexible, or is it bureaucratic? Can decisions be made quickly when necessary, or are they subject to a daunting hierarchy? Does the organization plan and adjust accordingly, or does it react abruptly? How does the organization communicate internally and with external stakeholders? Does the organization exceed the expectations of those it serves and those it employs? Do the organizations in the continuum have the same understanding of their respective roles? How do the roles of governance and management differ between organizations? Is one management team collaborative and focused on the success of the whole, while the other is competitive and focused primarily on the success of individual silos?

A clear understanding of the complexity of these "soft skills" and giving them appropriate weight in the decision to enter into the partnership will go a long way toward ensuring the success of the partnership or, if more appropriate, the decision to enter a partnership at all. Many of the other metrics of a successful partnership will not be achievable in the absence of cultural compatibility. Honestly acknowledging incompatibility and deciding not to proceed with a transaction will prove far less damaging to the organizations involved than discovering the misalignment after the fact.

Successful Partnerships

Experience shows that the critical factors for a successful partnership include the following:

- Articulation and mutual understanding of each partner's objectives and how they will be met (or not) by the proposed relationship
- Mutual statement of the vision, goals, measurable outcomes, and key milestones of the proposed relationship
- Understanding the needs and expectations of key stakeholders (including board, management, and staff), constituents, and community members regarding the benefits of the relationship

and the time frames for achieving those benefits
- Dedicated effort to engage and align the support of key constituents for the proposed relationship
- Discussion of obstacles, challenges, and potential pitfalls and the specific plans to address them
- Change-management process and communications strategy and dedicated resources to support the cultural change and implementation process ⊞

References

Booz & Company. 2013. "Succeeding in Hospital & Health Systems M&A: Why So Many Deals Have Failed, and How to Succeed in the Future." www.booz.com/media/uploads/BoozCo_Succeeding-in-Hospital-and-Health-Systems-MA.pdf.

Serota, S. 2013. "Insurers and Providers Integrating Toward a Common Cause." In *Futurescan 2013: Healthcare Trends and Implications 2013–2018,* 5–9. Chicago: SHSMD/Health Administration Press.

THE QUEST FOR AFFORDABILITY IN HEALTHCARE

by Bernard J. Tyson

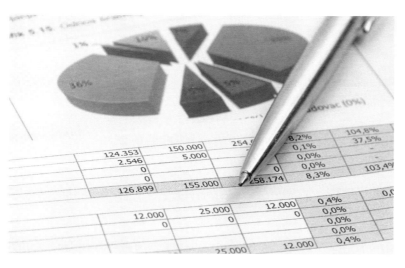

About the Author

Bernard J. Tyson is CEO of Kaiser Foundation Hospitals and Kaiser Foundation Health Plan, Inc. During his nearly 30-year career at Kaiser Permanente, which serves more than 9 million members in eight states and the District of Columbia, Tyson has successfully managed all major aspects of the organization. He has served in roles from hospital administrator to division president, leading Kaiser Permanente's business in California and other regions. In his previous position as executive vice president for Health Plan and Hospital Operations, he was responsible for both the care and coverage of members in one of the nation's largest health plans and hospital systems—38 Kaiser Permanente–owned hospitals and more than 600 medical offices across the United States. A San Francisco Bay Area native, Tyson received a bachelor of science degree in health service management and a master of business degree in health service administration from Golden Gate University in San Francisco. He earned a leadership certificate from Harvard University. He serves on the board of directors of the American Heart Association and as chairman of The Executive Leadership Council.

Healthcare in the United States is at a critical inflection point.

With healthcare costs expected to reach an unsustainable 20 percent of the country's gross domestic product by 2020, the entire industry is, rightfully, under intense scrutiny. The resulting transformation of the healthcare industry will require healthcare leaders to carefully consider revenue growth and cost management amid declining reimbursement for care.

There has never been a more exciting time to be in healthcare—or a more challenging one. We must look closely at one of our country's biggest and most pressing problems—the affordability of healthcare—and lead the way to solutions. Whether we approach the next decade with confidence or trepidation, one thing is certain: This is no time for business as usual.

The collective view of consumers, employers, and the government is that the cost of care is too high. As an industry, healthcare and its leaders need to be motivated to actively reduce costs and be prepared to face lower reimbursement rates that are intended to drive costs down.

Affordability will certainly be the dominant force for change in the healthcare market over the next decade and is one of the biggest drivers of the reimbursement trends discussed in this article. How we manage costs and continue to evolve our business models—while still delivering high-quality patient care—will determine our viability as we look ahead at the changing healthcare landscape.

Clearly, the new focus on costs will be long-term. Both in theory and in practice, organizations that own more pieces of the healthcare dollar can more effectively manage costs while maintaining high-quality standards of care. Certainly, moving to a bundled-payment approach—sharing more risk along the continuum—is intended to create greater efficiency and drive down the cost of care.

Other powerful currents of change offer potential solutions.

How likely is it that the following will be seen in your hospital's area by 2019?

Very Likely (%)	Somewhat Likely (%)	Somewhat Unlikely (%)	Very Unlikely (%)
48	42	9	1

Your hospital will have financial arrangements in place with physicians to support bundled payments.

How likely is it that the following will be seen in <u>your hospital</u> by 2019?

ACHE

27	38	27	7

SHSMD

40	43	15	2

Both

31	40	24	6

Your hospital will support a provider capitation model (receiving a set payment for members of the covered population for a period of time).

32	42	21	4

At least 15 percent of your hospital's patients will be under an at-risk (capitated) contract.

53	30	13	4

Your hospital will have made greater investments in alternate sites of care delivery (e.g., satellite outpatient facilities).

33	49	15	3

Your hospital will be financially sustainable with fewer inpatient admissions.

74	22	4	1

Your hospital's strategic plan will have a goal of reducing unnecessary admissions.

Note: Percentages may not total to exactly 100% due to rounding.

Organizations will support bundled payments. Nearly 90 percent of respondents think it likely that by 2019 their hospital will have arrangements in place with physicians in their area to support receiving bundled payments.

Hospitals will support a capitation model. Most survey respondents (66 percent of ACHE respondents and 83 percent of SHSMD respondents) predict that by 2019 their hospital will support a provider capitation model. Further, about three-quarters of survey respondents predict that at least 15 percent of their hospital's patients will be under an at-risk contract by that time.

Hospitals will invest in alternate care delivery sites. Most (83 percent) of the CEOs surveyed believe that by 2019 their hospital will have increased its investment in alternate sites of care delivery, such as satellite outpatient facilities.

Hospitals will be financially sustainable with decreased inpatient admissions. Among CEOs responding to the survey, 82 percent predict that by 2019 their hospitals will be financially sustainable with reduced inpatient admissions.

Strategic plans will target reducing unnecessary admissions. Almost all practitioners (96 percent) believe that their organization's strategic plan will, by 2019, include goals for decreasing unnecessary admissions.

Technology is mobilizing healthcare as never before, and the expectations of a younger, more diverse, and more sophisticated workforce demand innovation. We can harness this momentum to create a profoundly different healthcare delivery and financing system. But our true north should be our patients and customers, who deserve real value from new or revised ways of providing healthcare and services.

We must navigate to sustained improvement in healthcare in the United States, and I see the following trends shaping that journey.

Trends
Providers will shift from fee-for-service and volume-based measures to a provider capitation model, where risk and patient populations are managed differently than costs are. The current fee-for-service model, which rewards more use with more revenue, will go away in many markets. Enrollment in managed care plans has increased steadily since the 1990s, and this shift away from fee-for-service will accelerate as patients and purchasers recognize that more healthcare services do not

equate with better health outcomes (Kaiser Family Foundation 2012). The *Futurescan* survey results show that nearly 90 percent of hospital CEOs believe that by 2019 their hospital will have arrangements in place with physicians in their area to support bundled payments.

The rise of accountable care organizations and other pay-for-performance strategies is creating a demand for more transparency and is driving hospitals and physician groups to align and take on more risk as they struggle to improve performance and compete for market share. As a result, the healthcare industry continues to bustle with mergers and acquisitions, showing a 15 percent increase in activity in the first half of 2013 (de la Merced 2013). This receptivity to greater acquisition activity and partnership opportunities is reflected in the *Futurescan* survey data.

But managing costs is different from managing care, as we saw in the late 1980s and early 1990s when HMOs experienced tremendous public backlash because some plans were incentivizing physicians to restrict care and withhold services. Hundreds of plans either

closed or were acquired by competitors (Christianson, Wholey, and Sanchez 1991).

Successful risk-based models will keep central what is best for patients and will align payment incentives to promote value instead of volume of care. The *Futurescan* survey results indicate support for a provider capitation model by 2019.

Hospitals and healthcare systems will develop greater specificity around appropriate admissions. Hospital admissions for both government-sponsored and commercial populations have dropped significantly in many markets and are projected to drop in all markets over the next five to ten years (Grube, Kaufman, and York 2013). The trend of declining admissions is likely here to stay, as hospitals and healthcare systems adjust to declining reimbursement rates and revenue for inpatient services as well as new reform regulations that do not pay for hospital readmissions (for certain diagnoses).

Of the CEOs responding to the *Futurescan* survey, 82 percent predict that by 2019 their hospital will be financially sustainable with reduced inpatient admissions. And almost all (96 percent) believe that their organization's strategic plan will, by 2019, include goals for decreasing unnecessary admissions.

Hospital leaders will focus on wellness and prevention to further reduce preventable hospitalizations and to direct care to the right settings. Inpatient care will not be the default choice for care. Hospital leaders will have to provide more oversight of the appropriateness of care and apply care standards according to evidence-based medicine.

The treatment of routine back pain is a perfect example of how hospital leaders can influence adherence to best practices. According to a recent Harvard University study, many doctors are not following the established guidelines for care, which stress a less-is-more approach that includes core exercises, increased activity, and physical therapy (Mafi et al. 2013). Instead, physicians are exposing patients with back pain to unnecessary X-rays and potentially addictive prescription pain medication. They are also referring greater numbers of patients to specialists who are likely to perform spine surgery, despite little evidence that surgery is an appropriate first-line treatment for low back pain. If physicians consistently followed the established guidelines, patients would receive better and safer care, and hospitals could save payors a significant portion of the $86 billion annual cost of treating low back pain.

Hospitals will invest in alternative sites of care delivery and will develop a financial model that is sustainable with fewer inpatient admissions. Technology is changing the traditional footprint of care delivery so rapidly that it is hard to predict what the delivery model might look like in even five years.

Technology is making healthcare increasingly mobile and enabling patients to access care in convenient and customized locations, such as work sites and retail centers, as well as on mobile devices. As care becomes more mobile, patients' expectations around care and service will become more sophisticated. Savvier consumers mean increased expectations for connectivity and access. Decisions about where care is provided will be made from the patient's perspective instead of the provider's. New delivery configurations will have profound effects on hospitals' staffing and workflows. Consequently, hospital and healthcare leaders will have to champion new staffing and scheduling models that turn the old provider-centric paradigm on its head.

The acute care hospital will become the care setting for only the most critically ill, while outpatient care settings—enabled by technology—will provide preventive care and wellness, ambulatory, and post-acute care services in comfortable, customized, and convenient environments.

Hospitals will invest in technology, specifically electronic medical records (EMRs), to reduce the cost of care. Hospitals will invest in EMR systems to manage care for their patient populations, especially high-risk patients. In addition, hospitals will leverage EMRs to coordinate patient care—among the physician's office, hospital, laboratory, pharmacy, and patient's home—and to eliminate the pitfalls of incomplete, missing, or unreadable paper charts.

EMR technology offers caregivers immediate access to patients' critical medical information, resulting in better care. It also provides patients with access to convenient, time-saving features such as online scheduling, prescription filling, and

connecting with their doctors via secure e-mail.

Implications for Hospital Leaders

No matter where one lands on the payment continuum—bundled payments, shared risk, partial capitation, or full risk—assuming more risk will require healthcare organizations to invest substantially up front in the infrastructure for preventive care and care management and to tolerate longer payback periods on investments. This up-front financing could prove to be a barrier to infrastructure investment for small- to medium-sized healthcare providers.

Successful hospitals will empower physicians to manage care decisions and coordinate care throughout the continuum, including pharmacy, outside medical, post-acute, and end-of-life care and prevention and wellness services. Physicians will use real-time data to understand and manage the care of individuals, clinical cohorts, and communities. And they will practice evidence-based medicine, using proven clinical protocols to consistently yield the best care.

The increased emphasis on care management and quality will require leaders and organizations to be more interdependent than ever before. Vigilant oversight of transitional care is critical, and coordination of care will extend into the community as hospitals increasingly partner with community health advocates and other services to reduce admissions and address the social, economic, and behavioral drivers of hospital use.

With such phenomenal changes in the healthcare market, hospital and healthcare leaders have no choice but to seek new opportunities for growth while also driving greater affordability for consumers and patients. We will have to reinvent ourselves and develop new markets and niche industries to meet our patients' expectations for quality care that is also affordable. It will not be the biggest among us who will survive; it will be the most creative and resourceful. Bringing value to patients—focusing on our mission and not our margins—will drive innovation that leads to sustainable business in healthcare. As hospital leaders, we can be the solution that America deserves. ▣

References

Christianson, J.B., D.R. Wholey, and S.M. Sanchez. 1991. "State Responses to HMO Failures." *Health Affairs* 10 (4): 78–92.

De la Merced, M.J. 2013. "Merger Activity Was Down but Not Out in First Half." *The New York Times DealBook.* Published July 1. http://dealbook.nytimes.com/2013/07/01/merger-activity-was-down-but-not-out-in-first-half/.

Grube, M., K. Kaufman, and R. York. 2013. "Decline in Utilization Signals a Change in the Inpatient Business Model." *Health Affairs Blog*. Posted March 8. http://healthaffairs.org/blog/2013/03/08/decline-in-utilization-rates-signals-a-change-in-the-inpatient-business-model/.

Kaiser Family Foundation. 2012. "State Health Facts: Total HMO Enrollment." Published June. http://kff.org/other/state-indicator/total-hmo-enrollment/.

Mafi, J., E. McCarthy, R. Davis, and B. Landon. 2013. "Worsening Trends in the Management and Treatment of Back Pain." *JAMA Internal Medicine* 173 (17): 1573–81.

IT INTEROPERABILITY FOR CONTINUITY OF CARE

by John P. Hoyt, FACHE, and Michael S. Wallace, FACHE

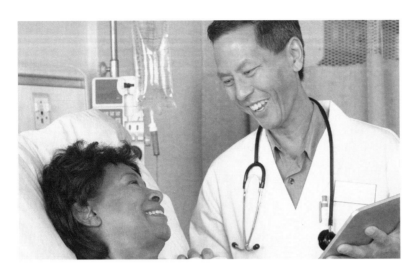

Why all the talk about continuity of care? What benefits can our industry gain from more coordinated care?

How broad should coordination of care be? What is the role of information technology (IT) in supporting continuity of care? How do today's CEOs view the future of care coordination and the governance and infrastructure required to achieve it? In this article, two executives address these questions from both a clinical care and an IT perspective.

What Is Continuity of Care?

For years, US healthcare has been delivered through partially coordinated silos that provide care on a one-on-one episodic basis—that is, a patient receives diagnosis or treatment from a different provider at each visit. For patients, this delivery

model has often resulted in the frustrating situation of having to repeat the same demographic information over and over to providers. In addition, the lack of coordinated care increases the potential for medication errors or excessive diagnostic testing because of the fragmented delivery system.

Coordination of care can be seen from two perspectives: the patient's and the provider's. From the patient's perspective, it can be described as a "continuous caring relationship with an identified health care professional" (Gulliford, Naithani, and Morgan 2006). From the provider's perspective, continuity of care can be defined as "the delivery of a 'seamless service' through integration, coordination and the sharing of information between different providers" (Gulliford, Naithani, and Morgan 2006). This latter definition makes reference to coordination among various providers, whether parts of a single corporate structure, such as an integrated delivery network (IDN), or a coordinated set of

About the Authors

John P. Hoyt, FACHE, FHIMSS, is executive vice president of HIMSS, a global, cause-based, not-for-profit organization focused on better health through IT. Before joining HIMSS, Hoyt served in senior management and chief information officer positions in various healthcare organizations and consultancy practices, including IBM Healthlink Services; Martha Jefferson Health Services in Charlottesville, Virginia; and First Data Health Systems Group. Hoyt holds a BS/BA degree in economics from Xavier University in Cincinnati, Ohio, and an MHA from St. Louis University in Missouri. He is a HIMSS Fellow and a Fellow and active member of the American College of Healthcare Executives. Michael S. Wallace, FACHE, is president and CEO of Fort HealthCare in Fort Atkinson, Wisconsin, an integrated delivery system serving a population of 85,000. He came to Fort HealthCare from Trinity Regional Health System in Rock Island, Illinois, and Bettendorf, Iowa. Wallace received his bachelor's degree from DePauw University in Greencastle, Indiana, and an MHA from the University of Pittsburgh. Wallace is board certified in healthcare management as a Fellow of the American College of Healthcare Executives (ACHE). He is the recipient of the ACHE Regent's Service Award and Early Career Healthcare Executive Award.

independent practitioners and hospitals. In addition, the providers' definition of coordination is

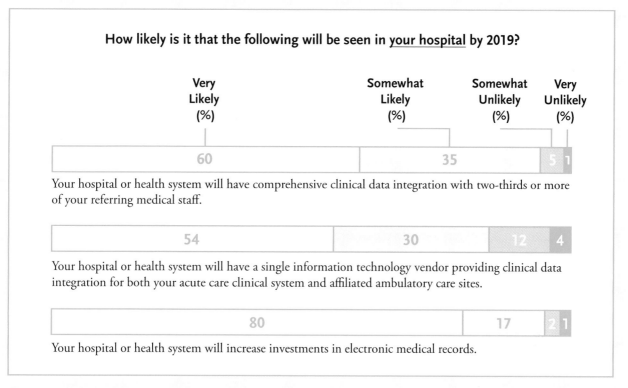

How likely is it that the following will be seen in <u>your hospital</u> by 2019?

Very Likely (%)	Somewhat Likely (%)	Somewhat Unlikely (%)	Very Unlikely (%)
60	35	5	1

Your hospital or health system will have comprehensive clinical data integration with two-thirds or more of your referring medical staff.

| 54 | 30 | 12 | 4 |

Your hospital or health system will have a single information technology vendor providing clinical data integration for both your acute care clinical system and affiliated ambulatory care sites.

| 80 | 17 | 2 | 1 |

Your hospital or health system will increase investments in electronic medical records.

Note: Percentages may not total to exactly 100% due to rounding.

What Practitioners Predict

Comprehensive clinical data integration will be in place. Most (nearly 95 percent) of the CEOs surveyed believe that their hospital or health system will have full clinical data integration with at least two-thirds of referring medical staff by 2019.

Hospitals or health systems will use one information technology vendor. Eighty-four percent of survey respondents predict that by 2019 a single information technology vendor will provide clinical data integration for their organization's acute care clinical system and its affiliated ambulatory care sites.

Investment in electronic medical records will increase. Of those responding to the survey, 97 percent think it likely that their organization will increase its investment in electronic medical records by 2019.

precisely the goal of the patient-centered medical home (PCMH) initiative. Key to the PCMH initiative is a robust exchange of health information among providers.

Support for Successful Continuity of Care

The principal benefits of coordinated care are quality and safety improvements. However, coordinated care also presents an opportunity for reducing diagnostic test duplication because clinical results can be shared among providers. Information sharing can take place through a robust private or public health information exchange (HIE) or through a single vendor. A single-vendor environment is not necessarily dependent on a complex HIE, which may be an investment beyond the financial or technical capabilities of small hospitals.

Continuity of care is not only for large IDNs—leading organizations of all sizes are pioneering care coordination supported by IT. Many of these organizations have developed strong partnerships with leading vendors that are able to serve both acute and ambulatory care with integrated clinical data architecture. Fort HealthCare, for example, uses a single-vendor model that supports the sharing of comprehensive medical information for coordinated care between acute care and ambulatory care providers. Fort HealthCare's inpatient facility is an 82-bed hospital with a medical staff of 100 providers.

Futurescan Survey Results

What do health system CEOs see happening in continuity of care by 2019? Will sufficient cooperation and incentives permit the development and maintenance of a comprehensive continuous care environment? Will IT investments support continuity of care? Let us look at some of the data from the *Futurescan 2014* survey.

Formal structure of care coordination. Of the CEOs surveyed, more than 85 percent think it likely that by 2019 most primary care physicians will support PCMHs as the best way to deliver value-based care (see pages 18–19). Further, 97 percent of the survey's respondents predict that within the next five years, their organization will participate in an HIE that allows sharing of health information among providers (see pages 6–7). But will sufficient incentives exist to promote coordinated care? Almost all (96 percent) of the survey's respondents agree that by 2019 incentives for their hospital and its associated physicians to deliver value-based care will be aligned (see pages 18–19).

Hospital viability with comprehensive care coordination. One consequence of comprehensive care coordination is a likely reduction in diagnostic services, which translates to a reduction in revenue for providers. Bundled payments will also likely result in a net reduction in revenue per care episode, necessitating care coordination to reduce the costs associated with delivery. Will IDNs be ready?

Almost 90 percent of the survey's respondents think it likely that by 2019 their hospital will have arrangements in place with physicians in their area to support bundled payments (see pages 28–29). Furthermore, 82 percent of the CEOs responding to the survey predict that by 2019 their hospital will be financially sustainable with reduced inpatient admissions, and almost all (96 percent) predict that their hospital's strategic plan will include a goal of reducing unnecessary admissions (see pages 28–29).

IT support for comprehensive care coordination. Do CEOs predict that hospitals and IDNs will invest sufficiently in IT to support comprehensive care coordination either through interoperability or a single-vendor approach? The future here looks bright according to the survey results.

Most (nearly 95 percent) of the CEOs surveyed believe that their hospital or health system will have full clinical data integration with at least two-thirds of referring medical staff by 2019 (see page 33). A mixed-vendor environment will likely continue through 2019, thus requiring comprehensive IT interoperability.

However, what is the likelihood that the complexities of HIEs can be minimized by a single-vendor solution for at least ambulatory and inpatient care? (In asking this question, we recognize that we are not considering potential integration with long-term care, public health, and other such care delivery environments; we stress ambulatory and inpatient care because they have the highest transaction volume.) A strong majority (84 percent) of survey respondents predict that by 2019 a single IT vendor will provide clinical data integration for their organization's acute care clinical system and its affiliated ambulatory care sites (see page 33).

Will investments in infrastructure and governance to support comprehensive care coordination result in efficiencies, enabling hospitals and IDNs to prosper under a bundled-payments program? Clearly, coordinated care can reduce prescribed medications and redundant testing. Prevention, wellness, and early detection initiatives will doubtless also mitigate the need for "downstream" services. Because the revenue streams associated with those services will be curtailed accordingly, coordinated care will be a critical component for providers in the evolving delivery system. Most (82 percent) of the survey respondents think their hospital or health system will reduce its ancillary costs, such as the costs of diagnostic or pharmacy services, by 10 percent per visit by 2019 (see pages 42–43).

With respect to electronic medical records (EMRs), practically all of the respondents (97 percent) expect to increase EMR investment over the next five years (see page 33). Fort HealthCare's experience corroborates this finding. Fort HealthCare's single-vendor integrated (ambulatory and hospital) EMR approach is reaping significant efficiencies for the organization. Anytime/anywhere access means the EMR can be viewed by more than one provider at any given time and accessed from virtually any computer with basic Internet connectivity. This accessibility can reduce the amount of ancillary testing that is unnecessarily duplicated. In addition, an integrated EMR facilitates best practices, standardizing care (reducing variation) within the community. Fort HealthCare now has one integrated record to document the health of its community.

Implications for Hospital Leaders

Comprehensive coordination of care, PCMHs, and bundled payments all call for IT support through HIEs or single-source clinical information systems.

Some leading organizations, small and large, have begun to derive benefits from coordinated care supported by robust IT infrastructure, such as single-source clinical solutions. "He who has the data will rule" will be the mantra of the future. More important, he who has the data and can turn it into meaningful information will be positioned for long-term success.

An IDN will be best positioned to succeed with a single comprehensive EMR, one that includes both acute and ambulatory health information for each patient. One way an IDN can effectively create an EMR is by partnering with a clinical software vendor that offers ambulatory and inpatient care in one product suite, one that has a common data architecture but does not require client-maintained interfaces. Market data show that of the hospitals and IDNs that switched from one core clinical vendor in 2011 to another vendor in 2012, 79.4 percent switched to one of three vendors—all of which offer ambulatory and inpatient care in one such product suite (HIMSS Analytics 2013).

However, as IDNs continue to acquire medical practices and subacute care institutions, the need for robust IT interoperability— through either a public or a private HIE—will continue until all the acquired practices and institutions are on a single product suite with a common data architecture and with vendor-maintained interfaces.

As medical practices approach the federal deadline for meaningful use, they will increasingly look to hospitals and IDNs to acquire them. Those practices that are not able to demonstrate meaningful use are likely driving down their own value.

Similarly, small rural hospitals that have not selected a comprehensive clinical vendor to enable continuous information flow for continuity of care are also probably driving down their acquisition value.

Much work remains to be done. But the race has clearly begun, and the early adopters are out ahead and beginning to reap the benefits of their investments in IT. ▣

References

Gulliford, M., S. Naithani, and M. Morgan. 2006. "What Is 'Continuity of Care'?" *Journal of Health Services Research & Policy* 11 (4): 248–50.

HIMSS Analytics. 2013. *Essentials of the U.S. Hospital IT Market: Applications of the EMRAM^SM*, 8th edition. Chicago: HIMSS Analytics.

ELIMINATING HEALTHCARE DISPARITIES: THE CALL TO ACTION

by Richard J. Umbdenstock, FACHE

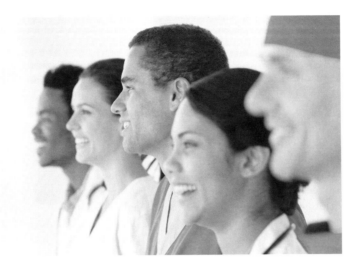

Racial and ethnic minorities now make up about one-third of the US population, but by 2042 they will become the majority.

While all patients are equal, they are not the same. They may, for example, be exposed to different environments and workplace hazards, have different diets, interact differently with healthcare providers, and face different challenges in complying with medical advice. For these reasons and many others, some still unknown, patients from traditional racial and ethnic minority groups often receive a lower quality of healthcare, even when the comparisons control for income and health insurance status (IOM 2003; Mayberry, Mili, and Ofili 2000). Healthcare disparities can lead to increased medical errors, longer hospital stays, avoidable hospital admissions and readmissions, and the over- or underutilization of procedures.

The REAL Challenge

Despite our best efforts, we know that race, ethnicity, and language preference (REAL) continue to affect the likelihood that patients will receive the care they need and the outcomes they deserve (IOM 2003; Mayberry, Mili, and Ofili 2000). For example, Hispanic adults with diabetes are far less likely to receive recommended preventive services, and African-American women are more likely to die after they are diagnosed with breast cancer, than are their white counterparts (AHRQ 2009; American Cancer Society 2011). As health insurance coverage expands, each provider will be challenged to provide the best possible care to a patchwork of patient populations with different beliefs, lifestyles, family structures and support, and healthcare experiences.

Planning for equitable care involves developing ongoing relationships with community organizations that can support providers'

About the Author

Richard J. Umbdenstock, FACHE, is president and CEO of the American Hospital Association (AHA), which leads, represents, and serves more than 5,000 member hospitals, health systems, and other healthcare organizations as well as 42,000 individual members. Previously, he was the elected chair of the AHA board. Umbdenstock's career includes experience in hospital administration; health system governance, management, and integration; association governance and management; HMO governance; and healthcare governance consulting. He has written several books and articles for the healthcare board audience and has authored national survey reports for the AHA and its Health Research & Educational Trust as well as for the American College of Healthcare Executives. He received a bachelor's degree in politics from Fairfield University (Connecticut) and a master's degree in health services administration from the State University of New York at Stony Brook. He is a Fellow of the American College of Healthcare Executives. He serves on the boards of the National Quality Forum and Enroll America, cochairs the Council for Affordable Quality Health Care (CAQH) Provider Council, and serves on the National Priorities Partnership and on the Center for Transforming Advanced Care steering committee.

efforts to build cultural competency in delivering that care. Providers must anticipate community needs to ensure access for those with limited or no English proficiency, for example, or to develop patient education materials that consider differences in both language and culture.

The use and types of measures of clinical quality and patient experience have increased significantly in recent years, and they are driving improvements across the board. But overall, national quality measures cannot be readily broken down by REAL. Recently, the Institute for Diversity in Health Management surveyed hospitals and found that although 81 percent of hospitals collect REAL data, only 18 percent have used those data for quality interventions (AHA and Institute for Diversity in Health Management 2012). Hospitals that collect accurate REAL data can begin to correctly identify their patient population. These data can also be used to break down quality outcomes by race and ethnicity and reveal if certain patient populations have lower-quality outcomes. Only at this level of data granularity can a hospital begin to implement quality interventions to reduce or eliminate disparities.

Call to Action

The need to address the problem of healthcare disparities led to the National Call to Action to Eliminate Health Care Disparities. In 2011, the American Hospital Association (AHA) stood in partnership with America's Essential Hospitals (formerly the National Association of Public Hospitals and Health Systems), the American College of Healthcare Executives, the Association of American Medical Colleges, and the Catholic Health Association of the United States to urge hospitals to speed up action to eliminate healthcare disparities. This was a bold but necessary step. To seek the field's support for action during a time of great change in healthcare was to acknowledge the urgency of improving equity of care.

The Call to Action focuses on three core areas that we believe will lay the foundation for all hospitals to reduce healthcare disparities:

1. increased collection of REAL data;
2. broader cultural competency training; and
3. diversity in governance and leadership.

Call to Action partners have set up the Equity of Care website (www. equityofcare.org) to help hospitals, healthcare systems, clinicians, and others improve the quality of care for each and every patient by sharing resources and best practices. We believe that most healthcare providers are moving in the right direction and that many are taking important steps to make care more equitable. But given the speed of change in our communities, we feel that this process must be accelerated and that information sharing is an important way to facilitate equitable care.

Call to Action partners recently set goals for each core area. By 2020, we hope to

1. increase collection and use of REAL data to 75 percent;
2. increase cultural competency training to 100 percent; and
3. increase governance and leadership team diversity to 20 and 17 percent, respectively, or to a composition reflective of the hospital's community.

For the field to achieve these goals and to sustain progress and momentum, hospitals need to make equity of care a priority and look beyond the immediate future.

Futurescan Survey Results
What are hospitals doing to promote equity of care? The Futurescan survey provides us with a view into hospitals' strategic thinking over the next five years. The majority (82 percent) of CEOs responding to the survey think it likely that goals for improving the quality of care for diverse

patient populations will be part of their organization's strategic plan by 2019. This is a key step for equity of care. We know that for real, meaningful change to occur, it must come from a hospital's leadership team. We also know that embedding key goals into a hospital's strategic process raises the issue to a level where results are seen. It becomes part of the work the hospital does and something to be believed in and integrated into its culture.

Understanding that disparities in healthcare are a problem is the first step toward achieving equity of care. Finding ways as an organization to reduce those disparities comes next. Again, we can look to the survey for an indication of what the future holds. Almost three-quarters of survey respondents believe that disparities of care among racially, culturally, and linguistically diverse patient populations will be reduced by half in their organizations by 2019.

Eliminating healthcare disparities is the ultimate point of the Call to Action and the goal of those who support equitable care. We do not have all the answers yet, but through the Call to Action and the Equity of Care platform, we are sharing resources and guides to help the field navigate toward high-quality care for all. To realize the goal of eliminating healthcare disparities, hospital leaders must believe that results can be achieved. The survey data highlight that this belief and commitment exist.

A hospital strives to reflect its community. As the demographic makeup of communities changes, hospital boards and leadership teams must change accordingly to reflect their community and align the hospital's work with the needs of a new population of patients. Call to Action goals around diversity address this movement and need for action.

How likely is it that the following will be seen in <u>your hospital</u> by 2019?

Very Likely (%)	Somewhat Likely (%)	Somewhat Unlikely (%)	Very Unlikely (%)
39	43	15	4

Your hospital's strategic plan will include goals for improving quality of care for culturally and linguistically diverse patient populations.

20	52	22	6

Your hospital will see a reduction of 50 percent in the disparities in quality of care among racially, culturally, and linguistically diverse patient populations.

ACHE

48	38	12	2

SHSMD

30	40	27	3

Both

43	38	16	2

The race/ethnicity diversity of your hospital board will represent your community.

ACHE

38	45	15	2

SHSMD

20	43	33	4

Both

34	44	19	3

The race/ethnicity diversity of your hospital's leadership team will represent your community.

Note: Percentages may not total to exactly 100% due to rounding.

Strategic plans will address diverse patient populations. The majority (82 percent) of CEOs responding to the survey think it likely that goals for improving the quality of care for diverse patient populations will be part of their organization's strategic plan by 2019.

Care disparities will be reduced by half. Almost three-quarters of survey respondents believe that disparities of care among racially, culturally and linguistically diverse patient populations will be reduced by half in their organizations by 2019.

Governing boards and leadership will reflect the community. A majority of those answering the survey (nearly 86 percent of ACHE respondents and 70 percent of SHSMD respondents) predict that by 2019 the racial/ethnic diversity of their board will reflect their community. Similarly, 83 percent of ACHE respondents and more than 63 percent of SHSMD respondents predict that the racial/ethnic diversity of the hospital's leadership team will represent their community by that time.

A majority of those answering the survey (nearly 86 percent of ACHE respondents and 70 percent of SHSMD respondents) predict that by 2019 the racial/ethnic diversity of their hospital's board will reflect that of their community. Similarly, 83 percent of ACHE respondents and more than 63 percent of SHSMD respondents predict that the racial/ethnic makeup of the hospital's leadership team will represent their community.

The governing board is crucial because it establishes the overarching direction of the hospital or healthcare system. A board whose makeup reflects that of its community has a far better chance of understanding its community's unique needs. This insight helps a hospital's leadership team strategically shift the approach to care, specifically in the area of equity.

Implications for Hospital Leaders

What does achieving equity in care mean for hospitals and healthcare systems? It results in better care and better outcomes, higher patient satisfaction, and a deeper and more meaningful connection to the community. Equity of care also has a strong business imperative; a study by the Joint Center for Political and Economic Studies found that eliminating healthcare disparities for minorities would have reduced direct medical care expenditures by $229.4 billion between 2003 and 2006 (LaVeist, Gaskin, and Richard 2009). As healthcare transitions to a value-based system of care, hospitals must ensure that their outcomes improve.

Hospitals can act immediately to address equity of care by developing consistent processes to collect and use REAL data. For example, they can ask patients to self-report their information and train staff, using scripts, to appropriately discuss patients' cultural and language preferences during the registration process. Hospitals should generate data reports stratified by REAL group to examine disparities. REAL data can be used to develop targeted interventions to improve quality of care (e.g., scorecards, equity dashboards) and can help create the case for building access to services in underserved communities.

In the area of cultural competency, hospitals should educate all clinical staff during orientation about how to address the unique cultural and linguistic factors affecting the care of diverse patients and communities and require all employees to attend diversity training. Hospitals should also provide culturally and linguistically competent services (e.g., interpreters, diverse community health educators) and features (e.g., a bilingual workforce, multilingual signage). In the area of diversity, a hospital should actively work to diversify its board and leadership team to include a voice and perspective that reflect its community. Accountability through the use of regular reporting on the racial and ethnic makeup of the leadership team will support actionable approaches. Diversification strategies include the creation of a community-based diversity advisory committee, engagement of the broader public through community-based activities and programs, and use of search firms.

The mission of the AHA and its members is to advance the health of individuals and communities. We are accountable to the community and committed to health improvement. We cannot succeed unless we eliminate healthcare disparities. As a partner in the Call to Action, we will keep the drumbeat steady and work closely with our members to foster success in the realm of equitable care. Equity in care is more than the right thing to do; it's the smart thing to do—for patients, for communities, and for hospitals.

References

Agency for Healthcare Research and Quality (AHRQ). 2009. *National Healthcare Disparities Report, 2008*. AHRQ Publication No. 09-0002. www.ahrq.gov/research/findings/nhqrdr/nhdr08/nhdr08.pdf.

American Cancer Society. 2011. *Breast Cancer Facts & Figures, 2011–2012*. www.cancer.org/acs/groups/content/@epidemiologysurveilance/documents/document/acspc-030975.pdf.

American Hospital Association (AHA) and Institute for Diversity in Health Management. 2012. *Diversity and Disparities: A Benchmark Study of U.S. Hospitals*. Published June. www.hpoe.org/Reports-HPOE/diversity_disparities_chartbook.pdf.

Institute of Medicine (IOM). 2003. *Unequal Treatment: Confronting Racial and Ethnic Disparities in Health Care*. Washington, DC: National Academies Press.

LaVeist, T.A., D.J. Gaskin, and P. Richard. 2009. *The Economic Burden of Health Inequalities in the United States*. Joint Center for Political and Economic Studies. Published September. www.jointcenter.org/hpi/sites/all/files/Burden_Of_Health_FINAL_0.pdf.

Mayberry, R.M., F. Mili, and E. Ofili. 2000. "Racial and Ethnic Differences in Access to Medical Care." *Medical Care Research and Review* 57 (Suppl 1): 108–45.

LARGE EMPLOYERS' RESPONSES TO HEALTHCARE REFORM: TRENDS AND OUTLOOK

by Helen Darling

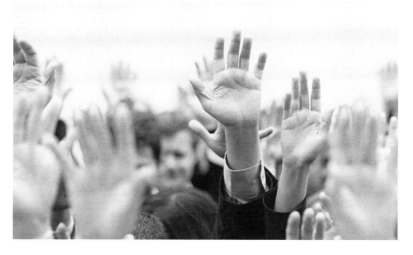

With a slow, nearly jobless recovery from the Great Recession, employers continue to be concerned about the costs of healthcare benefits for their employees and dependents.

Their concerns stem from the high cost per active employee (an average of $12,136 in 2013, up 5.1 percent from 2012) and the fact that this cost has increased much faster than wages (up only 1.6 percent per year for the past three years) (Towers Watson and NBGH 2013). In addition, healthcare costs have risen faster than both inflation and indicators of the economy's strength.

Macro Trends

The following macro trends have emerged among large employers as they address healthcare cost, safety, and quality:

- Spread of consumerism and consumer-directed or account-based health plans
- Increase in value-based plan designs
- Prevalence of comprehensive wellness and health improvement programs
- Demand for more transparency
- Promotion of narrow networks or direct contracting with centers of excellence, specialty centers, and accountable care organizations
- Promotion of primary care and medical homes
- Encouragement of employees to use a wide continuum of services that provides convenience, accessibility, and efficiency at lower cost (e.g., retail clinics, telemedicine, mid-level providers)

Healthcare reform has added to the healthcare costs of large employers in the form of new requirements, including dependent coverage up to age 26; the Patient-Centered Outcomes Research Institute fee; the reinsurance pool

About the Author

Helen Darling is president and CEO of the National Business Group on Health, a national nonprofit, membership organization devoted exclusively to providing practical solutions to its employer members' most important healthcare problems and representing large employers' perspective on national health policy issues. Previously, she directed the purchasing of health benefits and disability at Xerox Corporation for 55,000 US employees. The recipient of numerous awards, Darling received a lifetime appointment in 2003 as a National Associate of the National Academy of Sciences for her work for the Institute of Medicine. *Modern Healthcare* named her one of the 100 Most Influential People in Healthcare in 2011, 2012, and 2013 and one of the Top 25 Women in Healthcare in 2011 and 2013. In 2012, she received the Health Quality Leader Award of the National Committee for Quality Assurance (NCQA). She is chair of the board of directors of the National Quality Forum. She serves on the NCQA's Committee on Performance Measurement (as cochair for 10 years); the Medical Advisory Panel of the Technology Evaluation Center of the Blue Cross Blue Shield Association; the Institute of Medicine's Roundtable on Value & Science-Driven Health Care; the Medicare Evidence Development & Coverage Advisory Committee of the Centers for Medicare & Medicaid Services; and the Institute of Medicine's Committee on the Learning Health Care System in America.

How likely is it that the following will be seen in <u>your hospital</u> by 2019?

Very Likely (%)	Somewhat Likely (%)	Somewhat Unlikely (%)	Very Unlikely (%)
44	34	18	4

Your hospital or health system will develop or participate in narrow (e.g., "high performance") networks that provide a more limited choice of physicians and hospitals to health plans and consumers in return for net lower plan costs.

37	36	20	8

Your hospital or health system will contract directly with employers to offer packages of care for particular high-cost service lines (e.g., back surgery, selected cardiac care).

72	26	2	0

Your hospital or health system will make key information about your quality, safety, and efficiency (e.g., resource use) publicly available on a timely and regular basis in addition to HCAHPS reporting.

38	44	16	2

Your hospital or health system will realize a 10 percent savings in ancillary costs (e.g., diagnostic or pharmacy services) per visit from current costs.

27	37	27	9

Your hospital or health system will merge with other providers in order to reduce operating costs.

70	26	3	1

Your hospital will engage in process reengineering to reduce fixed costs.

Note: Percentages may not total to exactly 100% due to rounding.

Hospitals or health systems will participate in narrow networks. Of those surveyed, 78 percent predict that by 2019 their hospital or health system will develop or participate in narrow networks that offer net lower plan costs to health plans in exchange for a more limited choice of physicians and hospitals.

Hospitals or health systems will establish contracts with employers. Seventy-three percent of CEOs in the survey predict that by 2019 their hospital or health system will contract directly with employers to offer packages of care for selected high-cost services lines, such as back surgery or certain types of cardiac care.

Hospitals or health systems will report key information publicly. Virtually all (98 percent) of those surveyed believe that by 2019 their hospital or health system will routinely make key information about their quality, safety, and efficiency available to the public in a timely way.

Hospitals or health systems will reduce ancillary costs. Most (82 percent) of the survey respondents think it likely that their hospital or health system will reduce its ancillary costs, such as the costs of diagnostic or pharmacy services, by 10 percent per visit by 2019.

Practitioners are divided on mergers. A small majority (64 percent) of CEOs in the survey consider it likely that their hospital or health system will merge with other providers to reduce operating costs in the next five years.

Hospitals will reengineer to reduce fixed costs. Almost all of those responding to the survey (96 percent) think it likely that in the next five years, their hospital or health system will reengineer its processes to reduce costs.

tax; the elimination of annual or dollar limits on benefits; and a long list of new, poorly specified preventive services requirements.

Employers are eager to have more opportunities to select narrow, premier, or high-performance networks, although most are still interested in using plan design—for example, differential cost sharing—to encourage the use of in-network providers. Many employers are not ready to restrict their employees to narrow networks; however, the more evidence (e.g., provider performance data) that employers have to support network selection, the more easily they will be able to use plan design to promote high-performing providers. Respondents to the *Futurescan* survey clearly understand this trend, because 78 percent predict that their hospital or health system will participate in a narrow network. We can expect to see accelerated alignment in the next five years among employers, health insurers, and health systems.

Controlling Costs by Empowering Consumers

In the past four years, employers have become focused on a number of specific strategies and tactics for controlling costs. Employers believe that when employees have a financial stake in their use of healthcare services, they will use available tools and resources to make the best care decisions. As a consequence, more employers have been offering healthcare plans that entail higher cost sharing, including higher deductibles and coinsurance, instead of plans with flat copayments. These plans are generally referred to as *consumer-directed health plans* (CDHPs), *account-based health plans,* or *high-deductible health plans.*

According to a recent survey of members of the National Business Group on Health, approximately 72 percent of large employers now offer this type of plan (NBGH 2013). In 2014, 22 percent of employers will offer only CDHPs—that is, they will not offer any other plan types, such as an HMO or

traditional medical plans with low or no deductibles (NBGH 2013). Having only a CDHP often results in solid cost avoidance by employers and employees, depending on how much employers give to employees in the form of account contributions to offset higher deductibles. Some of the most experienced employers see CDHPs as a way to change the way employees think about their plans, how much healthcare they consume, and at what price—in short, to engage them as consumers (NBGH 2013).

Almost 79 percent of employers offer at least one tax-qualified, high-deductible health plan with a health savings account, while 26 percent offer a CDHP with a health reimbursement account (NBGH 2013). Evidence to date reveals that consumers in such plans use nurse advice lines more and visit retail or urgent care clinics slightly more than they do emergency rooms. CDHPs are especially appealing to those who use little healthcare. With evidence-based preventive care

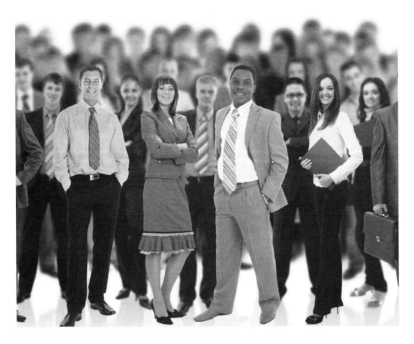

available at no charge to patients (not even as part of their deductible), low users of healthcare can save money. High users, especially those who take expensive drugs, will face higher initial costs until they meet their deductibles and out-of-pocket maximums.

Along with a plan that encourages consumers to become more engaged in the details of their care, employers reported that they buy a wide range of support services, most often from the health plan or insurance company that administers the self-insured plan. Eighty-four percent of employers pay for disease or care management; 69 percent offer decision support tools; 66 percent have a data warehouse and use analytical tools; 65 percent require prior authorization for selected services; 52 percent pay for health advocates or navigators for their employees and dependents; 29 percent offer second opinion services; and 28 percent use telemedicine (NBGH 2013). These services can provide a return on investment if targeted correctly and delivered efficiently. The fact that they are needed demonstrates how many problems exist

in our fragmented and complicated health system.

Transparency

In the past few years, transparency of information—such as data on charges, costs, efficiency, quality, safety, and patient experience—has become one of the most prominent challenges in the healthcare industry and one of employers' top priorities. Transparency is foundational if consumers and patients are to make choices that serve their best interests. Healthcare cannot come anywhere close to operating as an efficient market without trustworthy, meaningful information. Employers and other payors, including Medicare, have begun requesting or requiring data to inform their plan participants and to guide purchasing decisions. A growing number of major health plans (e.g., Aetna, Anthem, Cigna, Blue Cross and Blue Shield, United Healthcare) and third-party firms (e.g., Castlight, Change Healthcare) have websites and mobile apps that make quality data available and useful to consumers.

Some aspects of quality measures remain controversial—for

example, the fairness and effectiveness of quality measures at the level of individual doctors. But, however questionable accuracy and equity are, transparency will become the norm and the information available will improve accordingly. Hospital leaders appear to grasp the importance of transparency: 98 percent of *Futurescan* survey respondents believe that their hospital will make key information about quality, safety, and efficiency (e.g., resource use) and HCAHPS (Hospital Consumer Assessment of Healthcare Providers and Systems) data publicly available on a timely and regular basis. In addition to the 72 percent who consider it very likely, another 26 percent consider it likely.

Hospitals' and health systems' ability and willingness to share data on efficiency and resource use will expand as they engage in process reengineering to reduce fixed costs. Almost all (96 percent) of *Futurescan* respondents predict their hospital or health system will engage in process reengineering in the next five years. Most large employers are familiar with the power of business process reengineering methods, such as Six Sigma and Lean, and will welcome their use by health systems to reduce fixed and total operating costs.

With more transparency, employers and health plans will be able to use reference-based pricing as a tool to reduce costs and drive market changes. A recent study of joint replacement surgeries concluded that a California Public Employees' Retirement System (CalPERS) reference-based pricing benefit resulted in higher utilization of lower-priced facilities and lower utilization of higher-priced facilities, saving money for both CalPERS and its members (Robinson and Brown 2013). Employers will be eager to pilot more programs like this one.

Controlling Costs by Promoting Wellness

In surveys over the past few years, employers have reported that the main challenges to offering affordable health benefits are the poor health habits of employees and adult dependents (Towers Watson and NBGH 2011, 2012, 2013). High rates of obesity, sedentary lifestyles, and tobacco use increase medical and prescription drug claim costs. They also result in absenteeism, lower productivity, and "presenteeism"—when an employee is at work but underperforming for health-related reasons. According to a recent analysis, the fastest growing private-payor medical claims are related to musculoskeletal disorders, which are directly affected by obesity; complications of surgical and medical care; preventive care; and specialty drugs (Huse and Marder 2013).

Employers, other payors, and health plan managers see that they must reduce the demand and need for such care, and they plan to do so through programs and incentives that aim to identify and reduce risk factors that result in poor health and lead to serious illness and injury. Eighty-nine percent of large employers reported that they will offer tobacco cessation benefits in 2014; 88 percent will provide health assessments or health-risk questionnaires; 83 percent will offer biometric screenings; 77 percent will provide telephonic or on-site health coaching; and 55 percent will have on-site weight management programs (NBGH 2013). More and more employers are also requiring a health-risk assessment as a condition of access to the best health plan or health benefit package. The Affordable Care Act allows employers to offer incentives of up to 30 percent of the costs of the benefit plan to promote health improvement and wellness.

Implications for Hospital Leaders

Charges and transparency. Employers are worried that their healthcare charges will increase to offset unreimbursed charges of public payors, such as Medicare. As the percentage of patients covered by public payors expands, employers' fears will grow. Employers and their administering health insurers will seek ways to protect themselves—for example, through direct contracting; by offering narrow, high-performance networks; and by encouraging use of services and facilities not connected to hospitals. Employers and patients will seek out network providers that offer better contracted rates, and transparency will allow comparison shopping.

Patient cost sharing. As the prevalence of high-deductible health plans increases, more patients will not have the resources to pay their share of healthcare charges. Hospitals may get some relief from bad debt and charity care now that the newly created health insurance exchanges (HIXs) are online. States that have decided not to expand Medicaid are creating a pool of people who will struggle to afford cost sharing and even the modest premiums of HIX plans.

Performance. Employers and other payors will engage with narrow networks, high-performing networks, centers of excellence, or specialty units, sometimes through direct contracting. Employers will expect to benefit from increased efficiencies in the form of lower total charges and better results. For example, some savings may accrue to the employer and employee through faster patient recovery, fewer complications, fewer clinically unnecessary tests, and less rework. On the outpatient side, employers and other payors will want alternatives to emergency rooms, such as retail clinics. They will also want care options that keep people out of hospitals and away from hospital-based services. As hospitals try to provide a continuum of care to retain patients and capture revenue, employers and other payors will seek lower-cost alternatives.

Health and wellness. Employers' interest in health improvement and wellness could open up revenue opportunities for hospitals and health systems. Theoretically, hospitals may be in a good position to successfully promote health, especially to patients who have had a health event and thus have a strong motivation to improve. Millions of obese patients will need intensive outpatient counseling and related medical services. Hospitals, however, will need to bring their cost structure down to compete with fast-growing online and community-based services. Health systems may be able to offer clinically richer services, electronic medical records, care coordination, and benefits that other providers might not be able to supply. Given the cost pressures from all payors and the widening concern about how many services are unnecessary, redundant, or of no clinical value, more revenue and cost-per-unit problems could arise than ever before. ▣

References

Huse, D.M., and W.D. Marder. 2013. *What Are the Leading Drivers of Employer Healthcare Spending Growth?* Research brief, published April. Ann Arbor, MI: Truven Health Analytics.

National Business Group on Health (NBGH). 2013. *Large Employers' 2014 Health Plan Design Survey.* Industry comparison report, published August 28. Washington, DC: National Business Group on Health.

Robinson, J.C., and Brown, T.T. 2013. "Increases in Consumer Cost Sharing Redirect Patient Volumes and Reduce Hospital Prices for Orthopedic Surgery." *Health Affairs* 32 (8): 1392–97.

Towers Watson and National Business Group on Health (NBGH). 2013. *Reshaping Health Care: Best Performers Leading the Way.* 18th Annual Towers Watson/National Business Group on Health Employer Survey on Purchasing Value in Health Care. New York: Towers Watson.

_____. 2012. *Performance in an Era of Uncertainty.* 17th Annual Towers Watson/National Business Group on Health Employer Survey on Purchasing Value in Health Care. New York: Towers Watson.

_____. 2011. *Shaping Health Care Strategy in a Post-reform Environment.* 16th Annual Towers Watson/National Business Group on Health Employer Survey on Purchasing Value in Health Care. New York: Towers Watson.

Society for Healthcare Strategy & Market Development
  Executive editor: Don Seymour
  Executive director: Diane Weber, RN
  Managing editor: Mary P. Campbell

The Society for Healthcare Strategy & Market Development is the premier organization for healthcare planners, marketers, and communications and public relations professionals. A personal membership group of the American Hospital Association, SHSMD serves more than 4,000 members and is the largest organization in the nation devoted to serving the needs of healthcare strategy professionals. The Society is committed to helping its members meet the future with greater knowledge and opportunity as their organizations work to improve health status and quality of life in their communities. For more information, visit www.shsmd.org.

American College of Healthcare Executives/Health Administration Press
  Executive vice president/COO: Elizabeth A. Summy, CAE
  Director, Health Administration Press: Maureen C. Glass, FACHE, CAE
  Survey: Leslie A. Athey and Peter Kimball
  Project manager: Andrew J. Baumann
  Layout editor and cover design: Cepheus Edmondson

The American College of Healthcare Executives is an international professional society of more than 40,000 healthcare executives who lead hospitals, healthcare systems and other healthcare organizations. ACHE offers its prestigious FACHE® credential, signifying board certification in healthcare management. ACHE's established network of more than 80 chapters provides access to networking, education and career development at the local level. In addition, ACHE is known for its magazine, *Healthcare Executive*, and its career development and public policy programs. Through such efforts, ACHE works toward its goal of being the premier professional society for healthcare executives dedicated to improving healthcare delivery.

The Foundation of the American College of Healthcare Executives was established to further advance healthcare management excellence through education and research. The Foundation of ACHE is known for its educational programs—including the annual Congress on Healthcare Leadership, which draws more than 4,000 participants—and groundbreaking research. Its publishing division, Health Administration Press, is one of the largest publishers of books and journals on health services management including textbooks for college and university courses.

ABOUT THE SPONSOR

VHA Inc. is a national network of not-for-profit healthcare organizations working together to improve performance and efficiency in clinical, financial, and operational management. Since 1977, when VHA established the first hospital membership organization, the company has applied its knowledge in analytics, contracting, consulting, and network development to help members and customers achieve their strategic objectives. In 2012, VHA delivered $1.9 billion in savings and additional value to members. Serving 5,100 health system members and affiliates, VHA represents more than a quarter of the nation's hospitals. VHA also serves more than 118,000 non-acute healthcare customers enterprise-wide. VHA is based in Irving, Texas, and has 13 regional offices across the United States. VHA, together with UHC, owns Novation, a supply chain company, and its subsidiary aptitude™, the healthcare industry's first online direct market for contracting. VHA also owns Provista, a supply chain company serving the non-acute market as well as hospitality, education, and corporate markets. For more information, visit www.vha.com and follow us on Twitter (@VHAInc).

LEADERSHIP PRESENTATIONS AVAILABLE

Executive editor Don Seymour is available for on-site leadership presentations to healthcare governing boards, senior management, and medical staffs. To arrange for a leadership presentation, contact Mr. Seymour (617.462.4313 or don@donseymourassociates.com) or the Society for Healthcare Strategy & Market Development (312.422.3888 or shsmd@aha.org).